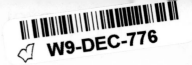

essentials of
pediatric
cardiology

essentials of pediatric cardiology

james h. moller, m.d.

PROFESSOR OF PEDIATRICS
UNIVERSITY OF MINNESOTA
MINNEAPOLIS, MINNESOTA

EDITION 2

 F. A. DAVIS COMPANY / PHILADELPHIA

Library of Congress Cataloging in Publication Data
Moller, James H.
    Essentials of pediatric cardiology.
    Includes index.
    1. Pediatric cardiology. I. Title.
RJ421.M56 1978   618.9'21'2   78-6306
ISBN 0-8036-6291-2

PREFACE

Since the writing of the first edition of the Essentials of Pediatric Cardiology many new developments have taken place. This new edition has been extensively revised and updated to reflect these changes and also incorporates the helpful suggestions of colleagues and students. As originally conceived, Essentials of Pediatric Cardiology still concentrates on presenting the major ideas and concepts of pediatric cardiology; in turn, I hope that students and colleagues will be able to apply these principles to effectively diagnose and manage new cardiac patients with varied or unusual cardiac problems.

Chapters 2, 3, 4, and 6 have been extensively revised and in some cases expanded. Chapter 2 contains new material on chromosomal abnormalities associated with congenital heart disease. The electrocardiography section (ECG) is now much more complete. Up-to-date information on echocardiography and other diagnostic techniques has been added. In Chapter 3, the discussion of cardiac abnormalities has been expanded to cover other congenital abnormalities as well. Chapter 4 discusses primary myocardial diseases much more extensively with added information on the prolapsing mitral valve and a separate section on cardiac arrhythmias. Chapter 6, Management and Treatment, now deals with such considerations as family counseling and bacterial endocarditis prophylaxis, in addition to more general material. I hope that these carefully planned revisions facilitate both the comprehension and usefulness of the essentials of pediatric cardiology.

I wish to thank my professors and mentors. I also wish to express my appreciation to my faithful secretary, Miss Mary Jo Antinozzi, for once more making the transition from completed draft to finished manuscript.

James H. Moller, M.D.

CONTENTS

1. **General Considerations** 1

2. **Diagnostic Methods** 3
   History 3
   Physical Examination 6
   Electrocardiography 23
   Thoracic Roentgenography 31
   Special Diagnostic Procedures 35

3. **Specific Congenital Cardiac Malformations** 45
   Hemodynamic Principles 45
   Acyanosis and Increased Pulmonary Blood Flow 50
   Obstructive Lesions 85
   Cardiac Conditions Associated with Right-to-Left Shunt 111
   Other Congenital Cardiac Anomalies 145

4. **Acquired Cardiac Conditions** 155
   Acute Rheumatic Fever 155
   Primary Myocardial Diseases 160
   Bacterial Endocarditis 165
   Marfan's Syndrome 167
   Prolapsing Mitral Valve 167
   Pericarditis 168
   Cardiac Arrhythmias 170

5. **Cardiac Conditions in the Neonate** 178
   Neonatal Physiology 178
   Cardiac Disease in the Newborn 181

6. **Management and Treatment** 185
   General Considerations 185
   Recommendations for Antibiotic Prophylaxis 189
   Congestive Cardiac Failure 191
   Cardiopulmonary Resuscitation 193

Index 197

1

GENERAL CONSIDERATIONS

With the advent of cardiac catheterization and angiocardiography, less emphasis has been placed on the more traditional methods of evaluating the cardiac patient. Most practitioners, however, do not have available to them these refined diagnostic techniques or the training to apply them. To evaluate the cardiac patient, the practitioner is therefore dependent upon either the combination of physical examination, electrocardiogram, and thoracic roentgenogram or the referral of the patient to a cardiac diagnostic center. Often the practitioner refers the cardiac patient to a center with the frustrated feeling, "Why should I make all these diagnostic tests and attempt a diagnosis when they will merely catheterize the patient?"

The purpose of this book is to formulate guidelines by which the practitioner, medical student, and house staff can approach the diagnostic problem presented by a child with congenital cardiac disease. Through proper assessment and integration of the history, physical examination, electrocardiographic findings, and thoracic roentgenogram, the type of congenital cardiac disease can be diagnosed correctly in 80 percent of the cases. Not only can a diagnosis be made, but the severity and hemodynamics of the anomaly can be correctly estimated.

Even though the patient may have to be referred for further study at a cardiac center, the physician will better appreciate the specific type of specialized diagnostic studies performed, and will better understand the approach, timing, and results of surgery. This book will help in the selection of patients for referral and offer guidelines for the timing of referrals.

The material is divided into five parts. *Diagnostic Methods* includes sections on history, physical examination, electrocardiography, and thoracic roentgenography. In addition, special procedures, such as echocardiography, cardiac catheterization, and angiography, are discussed. *Specific Congenital Cardiac Malformations* discusses the features of various cardiac malformations, and the principles previously discussed are applied. The anatomy and the hemodynamics of the malformations are presented as a basis on which to discuss the physical findings, electrocardiogram, and thoracic roentgenograms. Also, emphasis is placed on features that permit differential diagnosis of the various conditions. *Acquired Cardiac Conditions* presents three common cardiac problems affecting children: acute rheumatic fever, myocarditis, and paroxysmal supraventricular tachycardia. In addition, the cardiac manifestations of systemic diseases or conditions, such as hypertension, affecting primarily another organ system are described.

Cardiac Conditions in the Neonate describes the cardiac malformations leading to symptoms in the neonatal period and in the transition from the fetal to the adult circulation.

Management and Treatment presents the psychological and medical management of the child with a congenital cardiac malformation.

This book is not a substitute for the excellent texts of pediatric cardiology, but it should be used in conjunction with these texts as a guide to study and an aid to organization of thoughts and understanding of cardiology.

Certain generalizations will be made. In cardiology, as in all fields, exceptions occur. Therefore, not all instances of congenital cardiac disease will be correctly diagnosed on the basis of the criteria set forth here.

2

DIAGNOSTIC METHODS

The history, physical examination, electrocardiogram, and thoracic roentgenogram are the keystones of diagnosis of cardiac problems. By each technique, different aspects of the cardiovascular system are viewed, and by combining the data derived, a fairly accurate assessment of the patient's condition can be obtained. More sophisticated techniques such as echocardiography and cardiac catheterization permit more detailed patient evaluation.

HISTORY

The suspicion of a cardiovascular abnormality may be initially raised by specific symptoms, but more commonly the finding of a cardiac murmur is the presenting feature. Many children with cardiac disease are asymptomatic because the malformation does not result in major hemodynamic alterations. Even with significant cardiac disease the child may be asymptomatic because the myocardium is capable of responding normally to the stresses placed upon it by the altered hemodynamics. A comparable lesion in an adult might well produce symptoms because of coexistent coronary arterial disease or myocardial fibrosis.

In obtaining the history of a child suspected of cardiac disease, the physician seeks three types of data: 1) that which gives important diagnostic clues, e.g. cyanosis or squatting; 2) that which assesses the severity of the cardiac condition, e.g. dyspnea; and 3) that which suggests an etiology of cardiac disease, e.g. maternal rubella.

Children with cardiac anomalies may present with one of several cardiac symptoms or symptom complexes. The most dramatic of these, cyanosis, should be sought and its distribution noted. Cyanosis is a bluish or

3

purplish color of the skin caused by the presence of at least 5 gm/100 ml of reduced hemoglobin in capillary beds. The desaturated blood imparts a bluish color, particularly in areas with a rich capillary network such as lips or oral mucosa. The degree of cyanosis reflects the magnitude of unsaturated blood. Mild degrees of arterial desaturation may be present and cyanosis may not be noted. Usually, if the systemic arterial oxygen saturation is less than 88 percent, cyanosis can be recognized, although this varies with skin pigmentation, adequacy of lighting, and experience of the observer. A minimal degree of cyanosis may appear as a mottled complexion, darkened lips, or plethoric fingertips. Clubbing develops with more significant degrees of cyanosis.

Cyanosis is classified as either peripheral or central. Peripheral cyanosis, also called acrocyanosis, is associated with normal cardiac and pulmonary function. It is related to sluggish blood flow through capillaries so continued oxygen extraction leads to increased amounts of desaturated blood in the capillary beds. It typically involves the extremities and usually spares the trunk and mucous membranes. Exposure to cold is the most frequent cause of acrocyanosis, leading to blue hands and feet in neonates and circumoral cyanosis in older children. The cyanosis disappears upon warming.

Central cyanosis is related to any abnormality of the lungs or heart that interferes with oxygen transport from the atmosphere to the pulmonary capillary. Cyanosis of this type involves the trunk and mucous membranes as well as the extremities. A variety of pulmonary conditions, such as atelectasis, pneumothorax, and respiratory distress syndrome, can cause cyanosis because areas of the lungs while not being ventilated are perfused so that blood flowing through that portion of the lung is unoxygenated. Thus desaturated blood returns to the left atrium and mixes with fully saturated blood from the ventilated portions of the lungs.

Cardiac conditions can cause central cyanosis by either of two mechanisms. 1. Structural abnormalities divert portions of the systemic venous return (desaturated blood) away from the lungs. This can be caused by two categories of cardiac anomalies: a) conditions with obstruction to pulmonary blood flow and an intracardiac septal defect, e.g. tetralogy of Fallot, and b) conditions in which the systemic venous and pulmonary venous returns are mixed in a common chamber before being ejected, e.g. single ventricle. 2. Cyanosis of cardiac origin can develop from pulmonary edema. Mitral stenosis and similar conditions raise pulmonary capillary pressure. When capillary pressure exceeds oncotic pressure, fluid crosses the capillary wall into the alveolus. The fluid accumulation interferes with oxygen transport from the alveolus to the capillary so that hemoglobin leaving the capillaries remains desaturated. Cyanosis resulting from pulmonary edema may be strikingly improved by oxygen administration,

4

whereas cyanosis occurring with structural cardiovascular anomalies may show little change with this maneuver.

Congestive cardiac failure leads to the most frequently described symptom complex in children with cardiac disease. Infants with cardiac failure are described as slow feeders and tire on feeding, indicating dyspnea on exertion, the exertion being the act of sucking a bottle. The infant perspires excessively, presumably from increased catecholamine release. Rapid respiration, particularly when the infant is asleep, is an invaluable clue for cardiac failure in the absence of pulmonary disease. The ultimate diagnosis of cardiac failure rests upon a combination of information from the history, physical examination, and roentgenographic study.

Respiratory infections, particularly pneumonia, are frequently present in infants and less commonly in older children with cardiac anomalies, particularly those anomalies associated with increased pulmonary blood flow (as with left-to-right shunt) or with a greatly enlarged heart. The factors leading to the increased incidence of pneumonia are largely unknown but may be related in part to compression of the major bronchi either by enlarged pulmonary arteries or by an enlarged left atrium. Atelectasis may also occur, particularly in the right upper or middle lobe, in children with greatly increased pulmonary blood flow or in the left lower lobe in children with cardiomyopathies.

Squatting is a relatively specific symptom, occurring almost exclusively in patients with tetralogy of Fallot. When fatigued, cyanotic infants assume a knee-chest position, while older children squat in order to rest. In this position the systemic arterial resistance is raised, the right-to-left shunt is decreased, and the patient is less desaturated.

Dyspnea (labored breathing) is a symptom present in patients with pulmonary congestion either from left-sided cardiac failure or other conditions raising pulmonary venous pressure, or from marked hypoxia. Dyspnea is manifested in infants by rapid, grunting respirations associated with retractions. Older children complain of shortness of breath.

Fatigue on exercise must be distinguished from dyspnea as it has a different physiologic basis. Exercise intolerance of cardiac origin indicates an inability of the heart to meet the increased metabolic demands for oxygen during this state. This can occur in three situations: cyanotic congenital heart disease (arterial oxygen desaturation), congestive cardiac failure (inadequate myocardial function), and severe outflow obstructive conditions (inadequate cardiac output). Fatigue on exercise or exercise intolerance is a difficult symptom to interpret because other factors such as motivation or amount of training influence the amount of exercise an individual can perform. To assess exercise intolerance, compare the child's activities to those of peers and siblings, or to his previous level of activities.

Neurologic symptoms may occur in children with cardiac disease, particularly those with cyanosis, but are rarely the presenting symptoms. The causes of neurologic symptoms are discussed in subsequent sections.

Growth retardation is common in many children who present with other cardiac symptoms within the first year of life. Infants with cardiac failure or cyanosis show retarded growth, and the growth retardation is more marked if they coexist. Usually weight increase is more delayed than height increase. The cause of growth retardation is unknown but is related to inadequate caloric intake due to dyspnea during feeding and the excessive energy requirements of congestive cardiac failure.

Growth may also be retarded in children with a cardiac anomaly associated with a syndrome, such as rubella or Down's syndrome, which in itself causes growth retardation.

Developmental milestones requiring muscle strength may be delayed, but usually mental development is normal. In assessing growth and development it is helpful to obtain growth development data about siblings as well as the parents and grandparents.

Certain cardiac malformations have a definite sex predilection. Atrial septal defect and patent ductus arteriosus occur two to three times more commonly in female than male children. On the other hand, coarctation of the aorta, aortic stenosis, and transposition of the great vessels are more common in male children.

The age at which a cardiac murmur develops may give a diagnostic clue. The murmurs of congenital aortic stenosis and pulmonary stenosis are often heard in the neonatal period. Ventricular septal defect is usually first recognized at the 4- to 6-week examination. The murmur of an atrial septal defect may not be discovered until the preschool examination.

Other historical facts that may be diagnostically significant will be discussed in relation to specific cardiac anomalies.

A complete family history and pedigree should be obtained to disclose the presence of other congenital cardiac malformations, or other illnesses, such as rheumatic fever. The prenatal history may also suggest an etiology of the cardiac malformation if it yields information such as a history of maternal rubella or drug ingestion.

PHYSICAL EXAMINATION

When examining a child with cardiac disease, the physician may too quickly focus his attention on the auscultatory findings, overlooking the general physical characteristics of the child. In some patients these findings equal the diagnostic value of the cardiovascular findings.

Cardiac abnormalities are so often an integral part of generalized diseases and syndromes that recognition of the syndrome can often provide the clinician with either an answer or a clue as to the nature of the associated cardiac disease. Too often, medical specialists focus on specific body areas or systems, overlooking the forest of physical features.

In the following sections, diagnostic features of a variety of syndromes will be described briefly, with comments on the nature of the associated cardiac disease.

Syndromes with Gross Chromosomal Abnormalities

Down's Syndrome (Trisomy 21)

This syndrome has been found to involve complete or partial duplication of chromosome 21 in all or some (mosaic) of the body cells of the affected individual. The characteristics include slanted eyes, thick epicanthal folds, flattened bridge of the nose, thick protuberant tongue, and a shortened anteroposterior diameter of the head. The most common signs are short, broad hands, the short inward-curved little fingers, and a single transverse palmar crease (simian crease) together with a generalized hypotonia and joint hyperextensibility.

Cardiac defects are found in 40 percent of patients, with one third being ventricular septal defects, one third being endocardial cushion defects (usually the complete form of atrioventricular canal), and the remainder consisting almost exclusively of patent ductus arteriosus, atrial septal defects, and tetralogy of Fallot. It has been our experience that pulmonary vascular disease develops more rapidly in patients with Down's syndrome than in other patients with comparable defects.

Turner's Syndrome (XO or Gonadal Dysgenesis)

In this syndrome, there is complete or partial absence of one of the X chromosomes in all or some of the body cells in the female. The children have a female appearance but abnormal gonadal development. Characteristically they are short in stature, and have a stocky build, webbing of the neck, broad chest with widely spaced nipples, cubitus valgus, low hairline, and edema of the hands and feet (this can be a striking and diagnostic feature in newborns).

Cardiac anomalies occur in 35 percent of individuals with this syndrome, coarctation of the aorta being by far the most common defect (90 percent). Renal defects are common and may be associated with hypertension.

Turner's syndrome can be confused with the Noonan's or leopard syndromes (see below).

Trisomy 18 (E) Syndrome

Infants with an extra chromosome 18 have a low birth weight, multiple malformations, and severe retardation. Females live longer than males, but these children usually die within weeks or months. Overlapping of the flexed middle fingers by the second and fifth digits is very characteristic of this condition. Other features include micrognathia, low-set ears, rocker-bottom feet, umbilical and inguinal hernias, and generalized hypertonia.

Cardiac anomalies are present in over 90 percent of patients. In almost all, a ventricular septal defect is present, either as an isolated lesion or associated with origin of both great vessels from the right ventricle. Patent ductus arteriosus and bicuspid semilunar valves are commonly associated malformations. Pulmonary vascular disease frequently complicates the cardiac defect.

Trisomy 13 (D₁) Syndrome

Infants with an extra chromosome 13 have low birth weight and severe developmental retardation. Central facial anomalies, coloboma, and cleft lip and/or cleft palate are common. Microcephaly, prominent capillary hemangiomas, genitourinary defects, polydactyly, low-set ears, abnormally shaped skull, and rocker-bottom feet are other characteristic anomalies.

Cardiac defects occur in 80 percent of these individuals. The most frequent lesion is ventricular septal defect, but atrial septal defect, patent ductus arteriosus, and cardiac malposition commonly occur, often coexisting with the ventricular septal defect.

Syndromes with Familial Occurrence with No Evident Chromosomal Defect or Consistent Genetic Pattern

Noonan's Syndrome (Male Turner's, Ullrich-Turner Syndrome)

In very few cases of this type, sex chromosome abnormalities have been described. No specific genetic pattern has been found, though cases have been described in siblings and in successive generations. These patients typically show short stature, hypertelorism, low-set ears, and ptosis, presenting a rather characteristic facies.

The common cardiac defect in this syndrome is valvular pulmonary stenosis with thickened valve leaflets, but atrial septal defect and peripheral pulmonary stenosis may be present in addition. The electrocardiogram usually shows a superiorly oriented QRS axis (ranging around −90°).

Leopard Syndrome (Generalized Lentigo)

Patients with this syndrome show many of the features ascribed to Noonan's syndrome, but skin lesions and deafness tend to distinguish this syndrome from Noonan's. The term "leopard" derives from the complex of clinical features: multiple *l*entigines, *e*lectrocardiographic conduction abnormalities, *o*cular hypertelorism, *p*ulmonary stenosis, *a*bnormalities of genitalia, *r*etardation of growth, and sensorineural *d*eafness. In contrast to Noonan's syndrome, there appears to be a more consistent genetic pattern of dominant inheritance.

The cardiac defect tends to be similar to that in Noonan's syndrome— valvular pulmonary stenosis, either typical valvular or due to dysplastic valvular tissue. Subvalvular and supravalvular obstructive lesions have also been described.

As yet, there is no clear distinction between the two foregoing syndromes, and it is very likely that they represent the overlap of an array of distinct diseases. We have encountered instances of valvular pulmonary stenosis, with or without associated atrial septal defect, in siblings or in successive generations where the other physical features have been unusual but not characteristic of either of these two syndromes.

Supravalvular Aortic Stenosis Syndrome

This syndrome could be designated the "Alfred E. Newman Syndrome" in view of the resemblance of patients to this character in *Mad* comics. In some cases there is a clear-cut relationship to infantile hypercalcemic patients (earlier recognized as having a distinct and unusual facies), but others are sporadic and some follow a dominant genetic pattern. Again, it is likely that this syndrome encompasses patients of similar appearance but with etiologically different diseases. The physical characteristics include upturned nose with flattened bridge, long upper lip, cupid-bow mouth, full cheeks, prominent forehead, and brassy voice.

The characteristic cardiac defect is supravalvular aortic stenosis, but patients may also have peripheral pulmonary artery stenosis or systemic arterial stenosis as isolated or combined lesions.

Limb-Heart Syndromes

The association of congenital heart disease with deformities of the forearm was pointed out by Birch-Jensen in 1948. Subsequently, cases with deformities of the hand or forearm bones were designated as having the Holt-Oram syndrome (Holt and Oram having reported several cases in 1960) or ventriculoradial dysplasia.

Cardiac lesions tend to be atrial septal defects in the patients with carpal bone deformities and ventricular septal defect in those with a deformed radius.

There are certain diseases related to a gene-determined metabolic defect that lead to generalized signs and symptoms in which the heart may be

9

involved. Marfan's syndrome, glycogen storage disease Type II, and Hurler's syndrome are specific examples discussed in Chapter 4 (*Acquired Cardiac Conditions*), and their specific cardiac findings will be presented there.

Syndromes Following Infectious Disease

Rubella Syndrome

Maternal rubella infection in the first month or two of pregnancy commonly results in a newborn of low birth weight with multiple anomalies, the more striking being microcephaly, cataracts, and deafness. Hepatosplenomegaly and petechiae are among the other findings that may be present in infancy.

Cardiac defects are often present, with patent ductus arteriosus being the most common and peripheral pulmonary artery stenosis next in frequency.

Blood Pressure

In all patients suspected of cardiac disease, particular attention should be directed to accurately recording the blood pressure in both arms and one leg. This will allow diagnosis of conditions causing obstruction, such as coarctation of the aorta, recognition of conditions with "aortic runoff," such as patent ductus arteriosus, and identification of reduced cardiac output.

Many errors can be made in obtaining the blood pressure recording. The patient should be in a quiet, resting state, and the extremity in which blood pressure is being recorded should be at the same level as the heart. A proper-sized blood pressure cuff must be used because too small a cuff leads to false elevation of the blood pressure. Blood pressure cuffs of various sizes are available. The appropriate size for each age group is given in Table 1.

TABLE 1. BLOOD PRESSURE CUFFS

Age Group	Cuff Width
Infant	2" (5 cm)
1-5 years	3" (7 cm)
5-12 years	4" (9½ cm)
Older children and adults	5" (12½ cm)

Although a 1-inch wide cuff is available, it should never be used because it uniformly leads to a falsely elevated pressure. A 2-inch wide cuff can be used for almost all infants.

The cuff should be applied snugly and the manometer should be quickly elevated. The pressure should then be released at a rate of 1 to 3 mm Hg/sec, and allowed to fall to zero. After a pause, the cuff can be reinflated. Pressure recordings should be repeated at least once.

Three methods of obtaining blood pressure can be used in infants and children: the flush, palpatory, and auscultatory methods. In the *flush method,* used in infants, a blood pressure cuff is placed about the infant's extremity and the hand or foot is tightly squeezed by the physician's hand. The cuff is rapidly inflated and the infant's hand or foot is released. As the pressure slowly falls, the pressure value, when the blanched hand or foot flushes, represents the mean arterial pressure. In infants, blood pressure should be taken simultaneously in an upper and lower extremity because fussiness and crying can lead to falsely elevated values. This can be accomplished by connecting two blood pressure cuffs by a Y tubing to a manometer, placing one cuff on the arm and the other cuff on the leg, thereby obtaining the pressure simultaneously by the flush method. In infants it is easier to place the cuff around the forearm and leg rather than around the arm and thigh.

The *palpatory method* can also be used in infants. During release of the pressure from the cuff, the pressure reading at which the pulse appears distal to the cuff indicates the systolic blood pressure. A more precise but similar method uses an ultrasonic Doppler.

In the older child, blood pressure can be obtained by the *auscultatory method*: in the arm, by listening over the brachial artery in the antecubital space; or in the leg and in the thigh, by listening to the popliteal artery. The pressure at which the first Korotkoff sound is heard represents the systolic pressure. As the cuff pressure is released, the pressure at which the sound muffles and the pressure at which the sound disappears should also be recorded. The diastolic blood pressure is located between these two values.

The normal blood pressure values for different age groups are given in Table 2. The blood pressure in the leg should be the same as in the arm. Leg blood pressure should be taken with an appropriate size cuff, usually larger than the cuff used for measurement of the arm blood pressure. Since

TABLE 2. AVERAGE BLOOD PRESSURES IN CHILDREN AT REST

Age	Systolic	Diastolic
Newborn	60 (50-75)	35 (30-45)
Neonate	75 (60-90)	45 (40-60)
1-12 months	90 (75-100)	60 (50-70)
1-3 years	90 (75-110)	60 (50-75)
4-8 years	95 (80-115)	65 (50-75)
9-15 years	105 (85-125)	65 (50-80)

the same size cuff is frequently used at both sites, the pressure values obtained may be higher in the legs than in the arms. Coarctation of the aorta is suspected when the pressure is 20 mm Hg lower in the legs than in the arms.

Attention should also be paid to the pulse pressure. A narrow pulse pressure is associated with a low cardiac output or severe aortic stenosis. Pulse pressure widens in conditions with an elevated cardiac output or in an abnormal runoff of blood from the aorta during diastole. The former occurs in conditions such as anemia and anxiety, while the latter is found in patients with patent ductus arteriosus or aortic insufficiency.

Blood pressure must be recorded properly by listing on the patient's record the systolic and diastolic pressure values, the method of obtaining the pressure, and the extremity used.

In taking the child's pulse, not only the rate and rhythm but the quality of the pulse should be carefully noted, as the latter reflects pulse pressure. Brisk pulses reflect a widened pulse pressure, while weak pulses indicate reduced cardiac output. Coarctation of the aorta can be suspected by comparing the femoral and upper extremity pulses. Mistakes have been made, however, in interpreting the quality of femoral arterial pulses. Palpation alone is not sufficient either to diagnose or to rule out coarctation of the aorta. *Blood pressures must be taken in both arms and legs.*

The respiratory rate and respiratory effort should be noted. Normal values for respiratory rate are given in Table 3. Although the upper limit of normal respiratory rate for an infant is frequently given as 40 per minute, we have observed rates as high as 60 per minute in normal infants; the respiratory effort in these infants is easy. Difficulty of respiration is indicated by intercostal or suprasternal retractions or flaring of the alae nasae. Premature infants or neonates may show periodic breathing, so the rate should be counted for a full minute.

TABLE 3. NORMAL RESPIRATORY RATES
AT DIFFERENT AGES*

Age	Rates
Birth	30-60 (35)
First year	30-60 (30)
Second year	25-50 (25)
Adolescence	15-30 (15)

* Respiratory rates vary with changes in mental state and physical activity. Sleeping rates are slower and are indicated in parentheses. Depth of respirations and effort expended by the patient are equally or more important than the rate itself.

Cardiac Examination

Cardiac examination begins with inspection of the thorax. A precordial bulge may be found along the left sternal border in children with cardiomegaly. The upper sternum may bulge in children with a large left-to-right shunt and pulmonary hypertension or with elevated pulmonary venous pressure.

Several findings may be discovered by palpation, the most important being the location of the cardiac apex as this is an indicator of cardiac size. In infants and children under 4 years of age, the apex impulse should be located in the fourth intercostal space at the midclavicular line. In older children it is located in the fifth intercostal space at the midclavicular line. Displacement laterally or inferiorly indicates cardiac enlargement.

Thrills are best identified by palpation with the palm of the hand. Thrills are coarse, low frequency vibrations occurring with loud murmurs and located in the same areas as the maximal intensity of the murmur. In any patient suspected of congenital heart disease, the suprasternal notch should be palpated with a fingertip. A thrill at this site indicates a murmur originating from the base of the heart, most commonly aortic stenosis, less commonly pulmonary stenosis. In patients with patent ductus arteriosus or aortic insufficiency, the suprasternal notch is very pulsatile.

Forceful, outward movements of the precordium (heaves) indicate ventricular hypertrophy. Right ventricular heaves are located along the right sternal border, and left ventricular heaves are located at the cardiac apex.

Percussion of the heart in children is rarely worth the time required.

AUSCULTATION OF THE HEART

Auscultation of the heart provides perhaps the most informative diagnostic information, and should be performed in such a way as to obtain optimum information. A good stethoscope is a must. It should have short, thick tubing, snug-fitting ear pieces, and both a bell and a diaphragm. In most children, a ¾-inch bell and a 1-inch diaphragm are suitable for auscultation.

In infants, I initially auscultate through the clothing, despite the often quoted admonition that auscultation should never be performed in such a manner. Sometimes disturbing the child by removing his clothes results in a fussy state precluding adequate auscultation. Afterward, the clothing can be removed for another listen. Make certain the chest pieces of the stethoscope are warm.

In children between the ages of 1 and 3 years, it is easier to listen while they are sitting in their mother's lap, for children this age are usually frightened by strangers. In older children, physical examination can proceed as in adults.

When auscultating, I usually find it easiest to sit alongside the child. This position is neither fatiguing to the examiner nor threatening to the child.

Auscultation of the heart should proceed in an orderly, stepwise fashion. Both the anterior and posterior thorax are auscultated with the patient in the upright position. Then the precordium is reexamined with the patient reclining. Each of the four major areas (aorta, pulmonary, tricuspid, and mitral) is carefully explored. Both the bell and diaphragm portions of the stethoscope should be used in auscultation of the heart. High pitched murmurs and the first and second heart sounds are heard best with the diaphragm, while low pitched murmurs and the third heart sound are most evident with the bell. In auscultating the heart, attention is directed not only to cardiac murmurs but also to the quality and characteristics of the heart sounds.

Before we discuss the various heart sounds and murmurs that may be found on auscultation, the events and phases of the cardiac cycle should be reviewed. Figure 1 represents a modification of a diagram by Wiggers and shows the relationship between cardiac pressures, phonocardiogram, and electrocardiogram. In studying this diagram, relate the events vertically as well as horizontally.

The onset of ventricular systole occurs following depolarization of ventricles and is indicated by the QRS complex. As the ventricles begin to contract, the papillary muscles close the mitral and tricuspid valves. The pressure in the ventricles soon exceeds the atrial pressure and then continues to rise until it reaches the diastolic pressure in the great vessel, at which point the semilunar valve opens. The period of time from closure of the atrioventricular valve to the opening of the semilunar valve represents the *isovolumetric contraction period* because during this period blood is neither entering nor leaving the ventricles. During the next period, the *ejection period,* blood leaves the ventricles and the ventricular pressure slightly exceeds the pressure in the corresponding great artery. As blood flow decreases, eventually the pressure in the ventricle falls below that in the great vessel, and the semilunar valve closes. The pressure in the ventricle continues to fall until it reaches the pressure of the corresponding atrium, at which time the atrioventricular valve opens. The period between closure of the semilunar valve and the opening of the atrioventricular valve is the *isovolumetric relaxation period* because blood is neither entering nor leaving the ventricle.

Diastole is divided into three phases. The *rapid filling phase* comprises approximately the first 20 percent of diastole, and about 60 percent of blood flow occurs into the ventricle during this interval. The *slow filling phase* follows. Finally there is the period of *atrial contraction.* With the P wave, the atrium contracts and pressure rises slightly. An additional 15 to 20 percent of ventricular filling occurs.

14

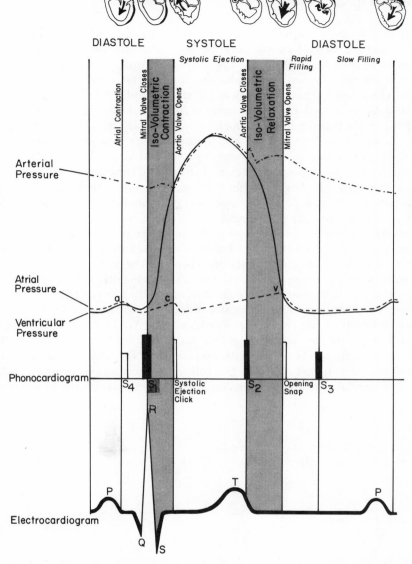

Figure 1. Relationship between cardiac pressures, electrocardiogram, phonocardiogram, and phases of cardiac cycle. S_1 = first heart sound. S_2 = second heart sound. S_3 = third heart sound. S_4 = fourth heart sound.

The timing and meaning of cardiac sounds and murmurs can be easily understood by considering their location within the cardiac cycle and the corresponding cardiac events. Although the origin of the heart sounds is uncertain, we will consider them to originate from valvular events.

HEART SOUNDS

The *first heart sound* represents closure of the mitral and tricuspid valves (Fig. 1) and occurs as the ventricular pressure exceeds the atrial pressure at the onset of systole. In children, the individual mitral and tricuspid components are usually indistinguishable, so the first heart sound appears single. Occasionally two components of this sound are heard. Splitting of the first heart sound can be a normal finding, although patients with complete right bundle branch block show wide splitting, since tricuspid valve closure is delayed because of delayed right ventricular activation. The first heart sound is soft if there is prolonged atrioventricular conduction, allowing the valves to drift closed after atrial contraction, or if there is myocardial disease. The first heart sound is accentuated in conditions with increased blood flow across an atrioventricular valve (as in left-to-right shunt) or high cardiac output.

The characteristics of the *second heart sound* are of great diagnostic significance in a child with congenital cardiac disease. The normal second heart sound has two components representing the asynchronous closure of the aortic and pulmonary valves. These sounds signal the completion of ventricular ejection. Aortic valve closure normally precedes closure of the pulmonary valve because right ventricular ejection is longer. The presence on auscultation of the two components, aortic (A_2) and pulmonic (P_2), is called *splitting* of the second heart sound (Fig. 2). The time interval between the components varies with respiration. Normally, on inspiration the degree of splitting increases, while on expiration it shortens. This variation is related to the greater volume of blood that returns to the right

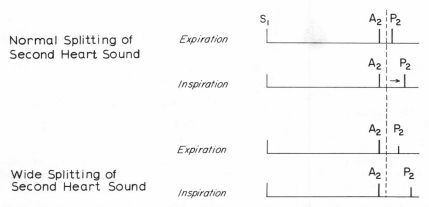

Figure 2. Respiratory variations in splitting of second heart sound. In a normal individual, P_2 (pulmonary component of second heart sound) is delayed on inspiration. Paradoxical splitting occurs in conditions delaying A_2 (aortic component of second heart sound). P_2 changes normally with inspiration. Thus, the interval between P_2 and A_2 narrows on inspiration and widens on expiration.

side of the heart during inspiration. Since ejection of this augmented volume of blood requires a longer time, the second heart sound becomes more widely split on inspiration.

Conditions prolonging right ventricular ejection lead to *wide splitting* of the second heart sound because P_2 is delayed further. This phenomenon is present in three hemodynamic states: conditions in which the right ventricle ejects an increased volume of blood (atrial septal defect), obstruction to right ventricular outflow (pulmonary stenosis), and delayed depolarization of the right ventricle (complete right bundle branch block).

Paradoxical splitting of the second heart sound is probably of greater importance in understanding the physiology of heart sounds than in reaching a cardiac diagnosis in children. Conditions prolonging left ventricular ejection may cause the aortic component to follow the pulmonary component (Fig. 2). Thus, as P_2 varies normally with respiration, the degree of splitting widens paradoxically on expiration and narrows on inspiration. Left ventricular ejection is prolonged in conditions in which the left ventricle ejects an increased volume of blood into the aorta (patent ductus arteriosus), in left ventricular outflow obstruction (aortic stenosis), and in delayed depolarization of the left ventricle (complete left bundle branch block). Thus wide splitting and paradoxical splitting of the second heart sound occur from similar abnormalities but on opposite sides of the heart. Paradoxical splitting is associated with relatively severe left-sided disorders.

In assessing a child with a cardiac anomaly, particular attention should be directed toward the intensity of the pulmonary component (P_2) of the second heart sound. The pulmonic component of the second sound is accentuated whenever the pulmonary arterial pressure is elevated, whether this elevation is related to pulmonary vascular disease or to increased pulmonary arterial blood flow. In general, as the level of pulmonary arterial pressure increases, the pulmonic component of the second heart sound becomes louder and closer to the aortic component.

The finding of a single second heart sound usually indicates that one of the semilunar valves is atretic or severely stenotic because the involved valve does not contribute its component to the second sound. The second heart sound is also single in patients with persistent truncus arteriosus because there is only a single semilunar valve.

A *third heart sound* is present normally in half the children and may be accentuated in pathologic states. This sound occurs early in diastole and represents the transition from rapid to slow filling phases. In conditions with increased blood flow across either the mitral valve (as in mitral insufficiency) or the tricuspid valve (as in atrial septal defect), the third heart sound may be accentuated. A gallop rhythm found in congestive cardiac failure often represents exaggeration of the third heart sound in the presence of tachycardia.

17

Fourth heart sounds are located in the cardiac cycle late in diastole, occur with the P wave of the electrocardiogram, and are synchronous with the atrial "a" wave. They occur in conditions in which the atria forcefully contracts when the ventricle has decreased compliance, as from fibrosis or marked hypertrophy, or when the flow from the atrium to the ventricle is greatly increased. The fourth heart sound may be audible, and if tachycardia is present, causes a presystolic gallop.

Systolic ejection clicks occur when the semilunar valves open and, therefore, mark the transition from the isovolumetric contraction period to the onset of ventricular ejection. Ordinarily this event is not heard, but in specific cardiac conditions a sound (systolic ejection click) may be present at this time and may be confused with a split first heart sound because of location in the cardiac cycle. Systolic ejection clicks indicate the presence of a dilated great vessel, most frequently from poststenotic dilatation. These sharp, high pitched sounds have a clicky quality. Ejection clicks of aortic origin are heard best at the cardiac apex, with the patient in a reclining position, and vary little with respiration. Aortic ejection clicks are common in patients with valvular stenosis and are less frequent in patients with coarctation of the aorta. Ejection clicks may also originate from a dilated pulmonary artery, as present in pulmonary valvular stenosis or pulmonary arterial hypertension. Pulmonic ejection clicks are best heard in the pulmonary area, with the patient sitting, and vary in intensity with respiration. Ejection clicks in patients with a stenotic semilunar valve occur more commonly in mild or moderate cases and may be absent in patients with severe stenosis. The absence of an ejection click in a patient with semilunar valve stenosis may therefore be indicative of a severe degree of stenosis. Clicks are not associated with subvalvular stenosis.

Opening snaps occur at the time the atrioventricular valves open. At this point the ventricular pressure is falling below the atrial pressure, the isovolumetric relaxation period ends, and ventricular filling begins. Ordinarily no sound occurs at this time, but if the atrioventricular valve is thickened or fibrotic, a low pitched noise may be heard when it opens. Opening snaps, rare in children, are almost always associated with rheumatic mitral stenosis.

MURMURS

Cardiac murmurs are generated by increased turbulence in the normal pattern of blood flow through the heart. Turbulence results from narrowing of the pathway of blood flow, abnormal communications, or increased blood flow.

Five aspects of a cardiac murmur should be noted that provide knowledge of the underlying cause of turbulence:

1. Location in cardiac cycle

2. Location on thorax
3. Radiation of murmur
4. Loudness
5. Pitch

Location in Cardiac Cycle

Murmurs may be classified by their location within the cardiac cycle (Fig. 3). A murmur is heard only during that portion of the cardiac cycle in which turbulence occurs.

Two types of systolic murmurs exist. *Pansystolic murmurs* start with the first heart sound and continue to the second heart sound, therefore encompassing the isovolumetric contraction period. Only three conditions permit blood flow during isovolumetric contraction: ventricular septal defect, mitral insufficiency, and tricuspid insufficiency. In the first, a pressure difference exists between the left and right ventricles throughout systole, while in the latter two the high pressure ventricle is in communication with the lower pressure atrium from the time of the first heart sound.

An *ejection systolic murmur* results from turbulent forward blood flow across either the aortic or the pulmonary valve. Since turbulent flow cannot begin until the semilunar valves open, an interval (the isovolumetric contraction period) exists between the first heart sound and the onset of the murmur. Although often diamond-shaped, systolic ejection murmurs are distinguished by the delayed onset of the murmur. Ejection murmurs are found in conditions such as atrial septal defect, aortic stenosis, and pulmonary stenosis.

Diastolic murmurs can also be classified according to their timing in the cardiac cycle. *Early diastolic murmurs* occur immediately following the sec-

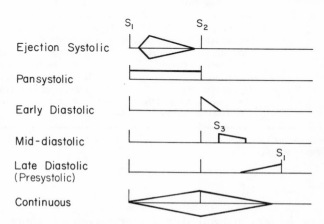

Figure 3. Classification of murmurs, showing location within cardiac cycle and usual contour. S_1 = first heart sound. S_2 = second heart sound. S_3 = third heart sound.

ond heart sound and include the isovolumetric relaxation period. During this time, blood can only flow from the higher pressure great vessel into the lower pressure ventricle. These murmurs indicate regurgitation across a semilunar valve (aortic or pulmonary insufficiency). They are usually high pitched and decrescendo. *Mid-diastolic murmurs* occur at the transition of rapid and slow filling pressure and result from increased volume of forward blood flow across a normal atrioventricular valve. In children, they most commonly occur with increased pulmonary blood flow and therefore increased blood flow into the ventricles. They are sometimes called an inflow murmur. *Late diastolic murmurs* represent organic obstruction of an atrioventricular valve. These murmurs are crescendo and low pitched. Rheumatic mitral stenosis is the typical example.

A *continuous murmur* indicates turbulence throughout the cardiac cycle. Usually this occurs when a communication exists between the aorta and the pulmonary artery or other portions of the venous side of the heart or circulation. Patent ductus arteriosus is the classic example, but continuous murmurs are present in other types of systemic arteriovenous fistulae.

The similarity between regurgitant murmurs and those due to forward blood flow, whether in systole or diastole, is summarized in Table 4. Regurgitant murmurs begin with a heart sound and include the isovolumetric periods, while those related to abnormalities of forward flow begin after an isovolumetric period and may be associated with an abnormal cardiac sound (systolic ejection click or opening snap).

TABLE 4. CHARACTERISTICS OF MURMURS

Location in Cardiac Cycle	Type of Murmur	
	Regurgitant	Forward Flow
Systolic	Pansystolic Begins with S_1; Includes isovolumetric contraction period	Ejection Systolic Follows S_1; Follows isovolumetric contraction period
Diastolic	Early Diastolic Begins with S_2; Includes isovolumetric relaxation period	Mid or Late Diastolic Occurs after isovolumetric relaxation period

S_1 = first heart sound.
S_2 = second heart sound.

Location on Thorax

The location of the maximal intensity of murmurs on the thorax provides information about the anatomic origin of the murmur. Auscultatory areas on the thorax have been described as: *aortic area* along the mid-left sternal border to beneath the right clavicle, *pulmonary area* along the upper left sternal border and beneath the left clavicle, *tricuspid area* along the lower left sternal border, and *mitral area* at the cardiac apex. For example, in these areas the murmurs of aortic stenosis, pulmonary stenosis, tricuspid insufficiency, and mitral insufficiency are found, respectively.

Radiation of Murmurs

The direction of transmission of the murmur is also helpful. Murmurs originating from the aortic outflow area radiate toward the neck and into the carotid arteries (valvular aortic stenosis). Murmurs from the pulmonary outflow area transmit to the left upper back. Mitral murmurs are transmitted toward the cardiac apex and left axilla.

Loudness

The loudness of a cardiac murmur is graded on a scale in which grade VI represents the loudest murmur. Conventionally, loudness is indicated by a fraction in which the numerator indicates the loudness of the patient's murmur and the denominator indicates the maximum grade possible (VI); therefore, grade I/VI would be very soft and grade VI/VI would be very loud. A grade IV/VI murmur is associated with a thrill.

Pitch

The pitch of the murmur can also be described as high, medium, or low. High pitched murmurs occur when there is a high pressure difference in the turbulent flow, such as in aortic or mitral insufficiency. Low pitched murmurs occur when there is a low pressure difference in the flow, as in mitral stenosis.

FUNCTIONAL MURMURS

Distinction between a functional (innocent) and a significant murmur can be a difficult problem in some children. Although in this text we will describe the characteristics of the commonly heard functional murmurs, only by experience and careful auscultation can one become proficient in distinguishing the functional from the significant murmur.

Functional murmurs have five features that help to distinguish them from significant murmurs:
1. The heart sounds are normal.
2. The heart size is normal.

3. There are no significant cardiac symptoms.
4. The murmurs are grade III/VI or less.
5. No thrill is present.

There are five types of functional murmurs. 1. *Twangy string murmur.* This is a low pitched, soft (grade I-III/VI) midsystolic murmur heard along the lower left sternal border. It derives its name from its vibratory character. Because of its location on the thorax it may be misinterpreted as a ventricular septal defect. It can be distinguished because it begins *after*, not with, the first heart sound as in ventricular septal defect. 2. *Pulmonary flow murmur.* This soft (grade I-III/VI) low pitched systolic ejection murmur is heard in the pulmonary area. The murmur itself may be indistinguishable from atrial septal defect. With this functional murmur, however, the characteristics of the second heart sound are normal; whereas in atrial septal defect the components of the second heart sound show wide, fixed splitting. 3. *Venous hum.* This murmur might be confused with a patent ductus arteriosus because it is continuous. It is, however, heard best in the right infraclavicular area. Venous hum originates from turbulent flow in the jugular venous system. It has several characteristics distinguishing it from patent ductus arteriosus: it is louder in diastole, is best heard with the patient sitting, diminishes when the patient reclines, and changes in intensity with movements of the head or pressure over the jugular vein. 4. *Bruits in the neck.* In nearly every child, soft systolic arterial bruits may be heard over the carotid artery and are believed to originate at the bifurcation of the carotid arteries. The bruit should not be confused with the transmission of cardiac murmurs to the neck, as in aortic stenosis. Aortic stenosis is associated with a suprasternal notch thrill. 5. *Cardiopulmonary murmur.* This sound originates from compression of the lung between the heart and the anterior chest wall. This murmur or sound occurs during systole, is loudest in mid-inspiration, and sounds close to the ear.

In most children with a functional cardiac murmur, neither a thoracic roentgenogram nor an electrocardiogram is indicated, as the diagnosis can be made with certainty from the physical examination. In a few patients additional studies may be necessary to distinguish significant murmurs from functional murmurs. The parents and the patient should be reassured of the benign nature of the murmur. No special care is indicated for these children, and they can be followed at intervals dictated by routine pediatric care. Most functional murmurs disappear in adolescence.

The abdomen should also be carefully examined for the location and size of the liver and spleen. The examiner should be alert to the presence of situs inversus. The hepatic edge should be palpated and its distance below the costal margin measured. If the edge is lower than normal, the upper margin of the liver should be percussed to determine the span of the liver. In patients with a depressed diaphragm (as from asthma), the liver edge is also depressed downward, and in this instance the upper extent of the liver is also depressed.

The spleen ordinarily should not be palpable. It may be enlarged in patients with chronic congestive cardiac failure or subacute bacterial endocarditis.

ELECTROCARDIOGRAPHY

Electrocardiography plays an integral part in evaluation of a child with cardiac disease. It is most useful in reaching a diagnosis when combined with patient data obtained from the history, physical examination, and thoracic roentgenogram. The electrocardiogram permits the assessment of the severity of many cardiac conditions by reflecting the anatomic changes of cardiac chambers resulting from abnormal hemodynamics imposed by the cardiac anomaly.

For example, left ventricular hypertrophy develops in patients with aortic stenosis. The electrocardiogram will reflect the anatomic change, and the extent of electrocardiographic change roughly parallels the degree of hypertrophy, yielding information to the clinician about the severity of the obstruction. A pattern of left ventricular hypertrophy, however, is not diagnostic of aortic stenosis because other conditions, such as systemic hypertension or coarctation of the aorta, also cause anatomic left ventricular hypertrophy and its associated electrocardiographic changes. Occasionally, electrocardiographic patterns are specific enough to be diagnostic of a particular cardiac anomaly, as in anomalous left coronary artery, tricuspid atresia, or endocardial cushion defect.

The electrocardiogram of children normally changes with age, the greatest changes occurring in the first year of life and reflecting changes in the circulation. At birth the right ventricle weighs more than the left ventricle because during fetal life it has supplied blood to the aorta by way of the ductus arteriosus and has had a greater stroke volume than the left ventricle. As the child grows, the left ventricular wall becomes thicker because systemic arterial pressure rises slowly, and the right ventricular wall thins as pulmonary arterial pressure falls. These anatomic changes affect primarily those portions of the electrocardiogram reflecting ventricular depolarization (QRS complex) and repolarization (T waves). Therefore, in infancy, because of the thicker than normal right ventricular wall, the QRS axis is directed more toward the right, and there are tall R waves in lead V_1 and deeper than normal S waves in lead V_6. With age, the QRS axis shifts into the normal range and leads V_1 and V_6 assume a pattern similar to that seen in adults (Fig. 4). In interpreting the electrocardiogram of a child, these changes and others that occur with age must be considered. Table 5 shows the range of normal values for several electrocardiographic intervals and wave forms.

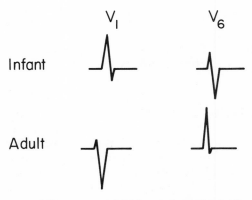

Figure 4. Comparison of the contour of QRS complex in leads V_1 and V_6 of infants and adults.

Analysis of an electrocardiogram should proceed in an orderly sequence to gain maximal information from the tracing.

The initial step should be to recognize any cardiac arrhythmias or major conduction abnormalities. These can usually be detected by the following three questions:

1. Are there P waves?
2. Is each P wave followed by a QRS complex?
3. Is each QRS complex preceded by a P wave?

If the answer to any of these questions is no, the type of rhythm disturbance should be further investigated by following the instructions given in Chapter 4.

The next step is to analyze each component of the electrocardiographic tracing. This is accomplished not by looking at each lead from left to right, as in reading a newspaper, and in so doing seeing the P wave, QRS and T

TABLE 5. NORMAL VALUES OF IMPORTANT ELECTROCARDIOGRAPHIC PARAMETERS

Age	QRS Axis (degrees)	R Wave in V_1 (mm)	S Wave in V_1 (mm)	R Wave in V_6 (mm)	S Wave in V_6 (mm)
0-24 hrs	137 (70-205)	16 (6-27)	10 (0-25)	4 (0-8)	4 (0-12)
1-7 days	125 (75-185)	17 (4-30)	10 (0-20)	6 (0-16)	3 (0-12)
8-30 days	108 (30-190)	13 (3-24)	7 (0-18)	8 (0-20)	2 (0-9)
1-3 mos	75 (25-125)	10 (2-20)	7 (0-18)	9 (2-16)	2 (0-6)
3-6 mos	65 (30-96)	10 (2-20)	7 (2-12)	10 (2-16)	1 (0-5)
6-12 mos	65 (10-115)	10 (2-20)	8 (2-15)	12 (3-20)	1 (0-3)
1-3 yrs	55 (6-108)	9 (2-18)	10 (2-25)	12 (3-21)	1 (0-3)
3-5 yrs	62 (20-105)	7 (1-16)	13 (2-25)	13 (4-21)	1 (0-3)
5-8 yrs	65 (16-112)	7 (1-16)	14 (2-25)	14 (6-24)	1 (0-3)
8-12 yrs	62 (15-112)	6 (1-16)	14 (2-25)	14 (8-21)	1 (0-3)
12-16 yrs	65 (20-116)	5 (0-16)	15 (2-25)	13 (8-20)	1 (0-3)

wave in each successive lead, but rather by reading up and down, first looking at the P waves in each lead, then looking at the QRS in each lead, and finally looking at the T wave in each lead. For each wave form, three features are analyzed: axis, duration, and amplitude.

P Wave

The P wave is formed by depolarization of the atria. Depolarization is initiated from the sinoatrial node located at the junction of the superior vena cava and right atrium. It proceeds generally inferiorly and leftward toward the atrioventricular node located at the junction of the atrium and ventricle, low in the right atrium and adjacent to the coronary sinus. The direction of atrial depolarization also proceeds slightly anteriorly. Since atrial depolarization begins in the right atrium, the initial portion of the P wave is formed primarily from right atrial depolarization, while the terminal portion is formed principally from left atrial depolarization.

The following three characteristics of the P wave should be studied.

P Wave Axis

The P wave axis indicates the net direction of atrial depolarization (Fig. 5). Normally the P wave axis in the frontal plane is $+60°$ ($+15°$ to $+75°$), reflecting the direction of atrial depolarization from the sinoatrial to the atrioventricular nodes. Therefore, the largest P waves are usually present in lead II and the P waves are normally positive in leads I, II, and aVF, always negative in lead aVR, and positive, negative, or diphasic in leads aVL and III. In the horizontal plane, the P wave axis is directed toward the left (approximately lead V_5). Therefore, the P wave in lead V_1 may be positive, negative, or diphasic.

The P wave axis is abnormal when the pacemaker initiating atrial depolarization proceeds differently from normal. One example is dextrocardia associated with situs inversus, in which the anatomic right atrium and the sinoatrial node are located in the left side, so atrial depolarization occurs from left to right, leading to a P wave axis of $+120°$ and resulting in the largest P waves being present in lead III. Another example is junctional rhythm, in which atrial depolarization proceeds from the atrioventricular node in a superior-rightward direction.

P Wave Amplitude

The P wave should not exceed 3 mm in height. Because most of the right atrium is depolarized before the left atrium, the early portion of the P wave is accentuated in right atrial enlargement. P waves taller than 3 mm indicate right atrial enlargement. This leads to tall, peaked, and pointed P waves, usually found in the right precordial leads or in leads II, III, or aVF.

25

P Wave Duration

The P wave should be less than 0.10 seconds in duration. When it is longer, left atrial enlargement or, much less often, intra-atrial block is present. Typically, in left atrial enlargement the P wave is broad and notched, particularly in leads I, aVL, and/or leads V_5 and V_6; there may also be a broad negative component of the P wave in lead V_1 because the latter part of the P wave represents principally left atrial depolarization, and because the left atrium faces the left precordial leads and the terminal P wave forces are accentuated and directed leftward.

PR Interval

The PR interval is the time from the onset of the P wave to the onset of the QRS complex. It represents the transmission of the impulse through the atrioventricular node and the Purkinje system.

The normal values of PR interval measured in leads I, II, or III are: 0.10 to 0.12 seconds in infancy, 0.12 to 0.15 seconds in childhood, and 0.14 to 0.22 seconds in adulthood.

Prolongation beyond these values is caused by prolongation of atrioventricular nodal conduction, as from acute febrile illness or digitalis. The PR interval may also be shorter than normal if there is an ectopic focus for atrial depolarization, as in junctional rhythm, or if there is an accessory conducting pathway into the ventricle with preexcitation, as in Wolff-Parkinson-White syndrome.

QRS Complex

The QRS complex represents ventricular depolarization. Ventricular depolarization starts on the left side of the interventricular septum near the cardiac apex and proceeds across the septum from left to right. Depolarization of the free walls of both ventricles follows. The posterior basilar part of the left ventricle and the infundibulum of the right ventricle are the last portions of ventricular myocardium to be depolarized. The QRS complex should be analyzed for the following three features.

QRS Axis

The QRS axis represents the net direction of ventricular depolarization. In children the axis varies because of the hemodynamic and anatomic changes occurring with age. The value of the QRS axis in the frontal plane for various ages is shown in Table 5. In neonates the QRS axis range is $+70°$ to $+215°$, but with age the axis comes into the range of $0°$ to $+120°$, most of the change occurring by 3 months of age. If the QRS axis falls within this range, the QRS axis is considered normal (Fig. 5). *Right axis deviation* is diagnosed when the calculated value for the QRS axis is greater than the upper range of normal, which for older children is more than $+120°$. Right axis deviation is almost always associated with right ventricular hypertrophy. *Left axis deviation* is indicated when the calculated QRS axis is less than the smaller value of the normal range. Left axis deviation is associated with myocardial disease or ventricular conduction abnormalities, such as occur in endocardial cushion defect, but it is rarely associated with left ventricular hypertrophy. When the QRS axis lies between $-90°$ and $-150°$ ($+210°$ to $+270°$), it is difficult to state if this axis represents marked right axis deviation or marked left axis deviation. In such patients, the physician should interpret the location of the axis, in light of the patient's cardiac anomaly.

Calculation of the direction of the mean QRS vector in the horizontal plane is more difficult, but it can be generally described as anterior, posterior, leftward, or rightward. Determination of the horizontal QRS axis can be combined with information about QRS amplitude to determine ventricular hypertrophy.

QRS Amplitude

In pediatrics, little diagnostic information is obtained from the QRS amplitude of the six standard leads except when low voltage is present in these leads. Normally, the QRS complex in leads I, II, and III should exceed 5 mm in height, but if smaller, the voltage is considered reduced and indicates conditions such as pericardial effusion.

In the precordial leads, QRS amplitude is used to determine ventricular hypertrophy. Leads V_1 and V_6 should each exceed 8 mm; if they are smaller, pericardial effusion or similar conditions may present.

Ventricular hypertrophy is manifested by alterations in ventricular depolarization and amplitudes of the QRS complex. The term ventricular hypertrophy is partly a misnomer, as this term is also applied both to the electrocardiographic patterns associated with cardiac conditions in which the primary change is ventricular chamber *enlargement*, and to patterns associated with cardiac conditions in which the ventricular walls are thicker than normal. Hypertrophy is the response to pressure loads upon the ventricle, whereas enlargement reflects augmented ventricular volume. An example of the former is aortic stenosis, and an example of the latter is aortic insufficiency.

Interpretation of an electrocardiogram for ventricular hypertrophy must be made in relation to the normal evolution of the QRS complex, particularly to the amplitude of the R and S waves in leads V_1 and V_6 (Table 5).

In right ventricular hypertrophy, the major QRS forces are directed anteriorly and rightward. This usually leads to right axis deviation, a taller than normal R wave in lead V_1, and a deeper than normal S wave in lead V_6.

Right ventricular hypertrophy can be diagnosed by either of the following criteria: 1) the R wave in lead V_1 is greater than normal for age, and 2) the S wave in lead V_6 is greater than normal for age.

A positive T wave in lead V_1 in patients between the ages of 7 days and 10 years supports the diagnosis of right ventricular hypertrophy. Patterns reflecting increase in right ventricular muscle mass ("hypertrophy") usually show an R wave in lead V_1, whereas patterns showing right ventricular enlargement usually show an rsR' pattern in lead V_1 and a qRs complex in lead V_6 with a large broad S wave. Usually the R' exceeds 10 mm. This distinction is by no means absolute, and variations occur.

In left ventricular hypertrophy, the major QRS forces are directed leftward and sometimes posteriorly. It can be diagnosed according to the following criteria: 1) R wave in lead V_6 is greater than 25 mm or greater than 20 mm in children less than 6 months of age, and 2) S wave in lead V_1 is greater than 25 mm or greater than 20 mm in children less than 6 months of age.

This may be combined with ST segment changes and inversion of the T wave in lead V_6, creating a pattern of "strain."

Distinction between left ventricular hypertrophy and left ventricular enlargement is difficult. Left ventricular hypertrophy may show a deep S wave in lead V_1 and a normal amplitude R wave in lead V_6, while left ventricular enlargement shows a tall R wave in lead V_6 associated with a deep Q wave and a tall T wave.

Biventricular hypertrophy is diagnosed by criteria for both right and left ventricular hypertrophy or by the presence of large equiphasic complexes in the mid-precordial leads with combined amplitude greater than 70 mm.

The electrocardiographic standards presented here are merely guidelines for the interpretation of the electrocardiogram. The electrocardiograms of a few normal patients may be interpreted as ventricular hypertrophy, and indeed with utilization of these standards, the electrocardiograms of some patients with heart disease and anatomic hypertrophy may not be considered abnormal.

QRS Duration

The width of the QRS complex should be measured in lead V_1. The normal range is from 0.06 to 0.10 seconds, with infants showing shorter QRS intervals. If the QRS complex is greater than 0.10 seconds, a conduction abnormality of ventricular depolarization is most likely present. Examples are right or left bundle branch block. In complete right bundle branch block, an rsR' pattern is present in lead V_1 and the R' is wide. The S wave is frequently broad and deep in lead V_6.

Q Wave

The Q waves should be carefully analyzed; abnormal Q waves may be present in patients with myocardial infarction. Normally the Q wave represents primarily depolarization of the interventricular septum. It can be exaggerated if there is infarction of the left ventricular free wall. After the initial 0.02 seconds of the ventricular depolarization, the left ventricular free wall begins depolarizing. With left ventricular infarction, the right ventricular depolarization is unopposed and directed rightward. This creates a larger and longer Q wave in the left-sided leads.

Q Wave Amplitude

Except in leads aVR, aVL, and V_1, the Q wave should not exceed 25 percent of the combined amplitude of the QRS complex. If it is larger, the initial QRS forces are accentuated, usually because of left ventricular myocardial damage.

Q Wave Duration

The Q wave in leads I, II, and V_6 should be less than 0.03 seconds. If the Q wave duration is greater, myocardial infarction is suspected.

ST Segment

The QRS complex returns to the baseline before forming the T wave. The segment (ST) between the QRS complex and the T wave should be isoelectric, but in normal children it may be elevated 1 mm in the limb leads and 2 mm in the mid-precordial leads. Alterations in the ST segment beyond these limits occur because of myocardial ischemia (depression), pericarditis (elevation), or digitalis (coving depression).

T Wave

The T wave represents repolarization of the ventricles. Whereas ventricular depolarization takes place from the endocardium to the epicardium, repolarization is considered to occur in the opposite direction. Thus, the direction of the T wave axis is in the same general direction as the QRS axis.

T Wave Axis

The T wave axis in the frontal plane is normally between $+15°$ and $+85°$ and in the horizontal plane it is between $-15°$ and $+75°$ (Fig. 5). Thus in the horizontal plane the T wave should always be positive in lead V_6. In V_1 the T wave is upright in the first 3 days of life and then is inverted until 10 to 12 years, when it again becomes positive.

When the T wave is not in the normal sector, the T wave is considered abnormal. If the QRS complex is also abnormal in showing either hypertrophy or conduction abnormalities, the T wave abnormalities are most likely secondary to the QRS changes. If, however, the QRS complex is normal, the T wave changes are considered primary and may be caused by a variety of factors, such as electrolyte abnormality.

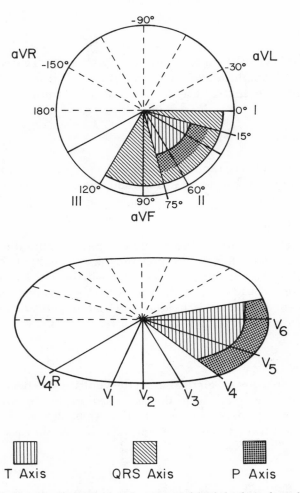

Figure 5. Relationship of standard and augmented limb leads in frontal plane (above) and precordial leads in horizontal plane (below). The normal ranges for the P wave, QRS complex, and T wave axes in frontal plane and the P and T wave axes in horizontal plane are shown.

T Wave Amplitude

There are no rigid criteria for the amplitude of T waves, although generally the greater the amplitude of the QRS, the greater the T wave. The T waves normally range from 1 to 5 mm in standard leads and from 2 to 8 mm in precordial leads.

The T wave amplitude is also affected by serum potassium concentration. Hypokalemia is associated by low voltage T waves, and hyperkalemia is associated by tall, peaked, and *symmetrical* T waves.

T Wave Duration

This is best measured by the QT interval: the time from onset of the Q wave to termination of the T wave. Since this is variable naturally with heart rate, it needs to be corrected—

$$QTc = \frac{QT}{\sqrt{R\text{-}R}}$$

The QTc normally is 0.38 seconds. Hypercalcemia and digitalis shorten the QTc and hypocalcemia lengthens it.

U Wave

Finally, in some patients a small deflection of unknown origin, the U wave, follows the T wave. It is of no diagnostic significance, although it may be prominent in patients with hypokalemia.

The electrocardiogram can also be used to detect cardiac arrhythmias or conduction abnormalities. The most important of these rhythm disturbances are discussed in Chapter 4.

THORACIC ROENTGENOGRAPHY

Thoracic roentgenograms should be made on every patient suspected of cardiac disease. Study of the x-ray films reveals information about: the cardiac size, the size of specific cardiac chambers, the status of the pulmonary vasculature, and the variations of cardiac contour. To gain this type of information, four views of the heart are usually obtained, these being posteroanterior, lateral, left anterior oblique, and right anterior oblique. A barium swallow is obtained with each film, since the barium-filled esophagus aids in visualization of cardiac structures.

Cardiac size can be evaluated best on a posteroanterior projection. Cardiac enlargement indicates augmented volume of blood in the heart. Any condition that places a volume load upon the heart, as from an insufficient valve or a left-to-right shunt, leads to cardiac enlargement proportional to the amount of volume overload. In contrast, ventricular hypertrophy, meaning increased thickness of the myocardium, does not show as cardiac enlargement on the roentgenogram, although it might change the contour of the heart. *Cardiac enlargement means increased volume of blood in the heart.*

Specific cardiac chamber size is best evaluated by interpretation of the four views of the heart. The anatomic position of the cardiac chambers in each of the four views is shown in Figure 6. Several important anatomic features are illustrated. The atria and ventricles, rather than being positioned in true right-to-left relationship, have a more anteroposterior orientation. The right atrium and right ventricle are anterior and to the right of the respective left-sided chambers. The interatrial and interventricular septae are not perpendicular to the anterior chest wall but are at a 45° angle to the left.

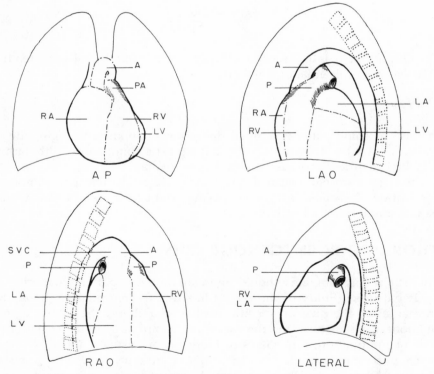

Figure 6. Relationship of cardiac chambers observed in four roentgenographic views of the heart. A = aorta. AP = anteroposterior. LA = left atrium. LAO = left anterior oblique. LV = left ventricle. P, PA = pulmonary artery. RA = right atrium. RAO = right anterior oblique and lateral. RV = right ventricle. SVC = superior vena cava.

In the posteroanterior projection, the right cardiac border is formed by the right atrium. Prominence of this cardiac border may suggest right atrial enlargement, but this diagnosis is difficult to make definitely from the roentgenogram. The left cardiac border is composed of three segments: the aortic knob, pulmonary trunk, and broad sweep of the left ventricle. The right ventricle is not seen on this projection.

Prominence of the aorta or the pulmonary trunk may be found on this view. Enlargement of either of these vessels occurs in any of three hemodynamic situations: increased blood flow through the great vessel, poststenotic dilatation, or increased pressure beyond the valve, as in pulmonary hypertension. A concave pulmonary arterial segment indicates diminished volume of pulmonary blood flow.

On the lateral film the margins of the cardiac silhouette are formed anteriorly by the right ventricle and posteriorly by the left atrium. This is the preferred view for showing left atrial enlargement because the left atrium is the only cardiac chamber that normally touches the esophagus. In normal individuals, the left atrium may indent the anterior wall, but the posterior wall is not displaced. If both anterior and posterior walls are displaced, left atrial enlargement is present. Normally, the air-filled lung extends down between the sternum and the right ventricle. When the retrosternal space is obliterated by cardiac density, right ventricular enlargement is present, although in infants this space may also be obliterated by the thymus.

In the left anterior oblique projection, the x-ray picture is taken with the patient turned 45° to the right. Thus, in this view the heart is positioned so that the interventricular septum is in the middle of the cardiac silhouette. The right ventricle lies anteriorly and the left ventricle lies posteriorly. Left ventricular enlargement may be detected on this view by the extension of the cardiac apex inferiorly and leftward.

In the right anterior oblique projection, the heart is viewed from a 60° angle to the right of the midline; this projection yields information similar to that of the lateral view, although the pulmonary conus is brought out better. The right ventricle and the pulmonary conus are located anteriorly, and the left atrium is posteriorly positioned in relation to the esophagus. Right ventricular enlargement is evident as a prominent anterior bulge, while left atrial enlargement shows a displacement of the esophagus.

Both the electrocardiogram and the thoracic roentgenogram may be used to assess cardiac chamber size. Left atrial enlargement is best detected by thoracic roentgenogram, while ventricular or right atrial enlargement is better detected by electrocardiogram.

The status of the pulmonary vasculature is the most important diagnostic information derived from the thoracic roentgenogram. The roentgenographic appearance of the blood vessels in the lungs reflects the volume of pulmonary blood flow. Because many cardiac anomalies alter pulmonary blood flow, proper interpretation of pulmonary vascular markings is diagnostically helpful. It is one of the two major features in initiating the differential diagnosis discussed in this book.

The lung fields are assessed to determine if the vascularity is increased, normal, or diminished, reflecting augmented, normal, or decreased volume of pulmonary blood flow, respectively. As a check on the logic of interpretation, the vascular markings should be compared with cardiac

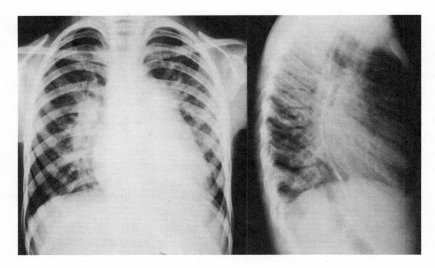

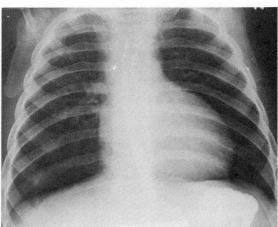

Figure 7. Roentgenographic appearance of pulmonary vasculature. Top. Increased pulmonary vascular markings in a patient with ventricular septal defect. Also, posterior displacement of barium-filled esophagus by enlarged left atrium on lateral view (right). Bottom. Decreased pulmonary vascular markings in a patient with tricuspid atresia.

size. If there is a large volume left-to-right shunt, the volume of the heart will necessarily be larger than normal.

On the basis of experience obtained from viewing a number of thoracic roentgenograms, the status of pulmonary vasculature can be judged. Examples of increased and decreased vascularity are shown in Figure 7. In the former, the lung fields show increased pulmonary arterial markings, the hilum is plump, and vascular shadows radiate to the periphery. With decreased vascularity, the lungs appear dark or lucent, the hilum is small, and the pulmonary arterial vessels are stringy.

In addition to the search for information about cardiac size on the posteroanterior view of the heart, attention is directed to distinctive cardiac contours, such as the boot-shaped heart of tetralogy of Fallot. In conditions with right ventricular hypertrophy, the cardiac apex may be turned upward, while conditions with left ventricular hypertrophy or dilatation lead to displacement of the cardiac apex outward and downward toward the diaphragm.

SPECIAL DIAGNOSTIC PROCEDURES

Aside from the four traditional methods of evaluating cardiac status, there are other procedures yielding information that may help solve diagnostic or therapeutic problems.

Hemoglobin and Hematocrit Determinations

In infants and children with cyanotic forms of congenital cardiac disease, the hypoxia stimulates the bone marrow to produce an increased number of red blood cells. Oxygen carrying capacity is thereby improved. As a result both the total number of erythrocytes and the hematocrit are elevated. The production of the increased red cell mass should be paralleled by an increase in hemoglobin. In a patient with cyanosis and normal iron stores, the hemoglobin should also be elevated so that the red cell indices are normal.

In infancy, however, iron deficiency is common and may be accentuated in cyanotic infants because of the increased iron requirements and the fact that such infants may have poor appetites and primarily a milk diet. In such infants the red cell indices reflect iron deficiency anemia because the hemoglobin value is low in relation to the red blood count and the hematocrit. In fact, a cyanotic infant may have a hemoglobin value that is normal or even elevated for age and still have iron deficiency. An example would be an infant with a hemoglobin of 16 gm/100 ml and a hematocrit of 66 percent. The hematocrit value reflects the volume of red cells that are elevated in response to hypoxia, while the hemoglobin value reflects primarily the amount of iron available for its formation. In this infant the hemoglobin should be 22 gm/100 ml (normally the number for the hemoglobin value should be one third that of the number of the hematocrit value). An iron-deficient infant requires the administration of iron; his symptoms may improve dramatically following such treatment.

Patients with cyanotic heart disease should have hemoglobin and hematocrit values obtained periodically. Similar information might be obtained by evaluating a blood smear. Determination of serum iron is usually not necessary.

Echocardiography

Ultrasonography is a diagnostic technique that has recently been applied to cardiology. As echocardiography, this method adds considerable information regarding cardiac function and structure. The knowledge and concepts of echocardiography will increase with time and the applications and specificity of this technique become better defined. Most cardiac centers now perform echocardiography; in the diagnostic evaluation of a patient, it ranks with thoracic roentgenography and electrocardiography. It also has the advantage of being a noninvasive technique.

Echocardiography is based on a familiar principle illustrated by birds and certain animals, such as bats, that emit ultrahigh frequency sound waves. These sound waves are reflected from surfaces and are received back, allowing the bats to judge their surroundings and to avoid collision with objects. This principle has been applied to oceanography and subsequently used for submarine detection. During the last few years, ultrasonography has been used in many areas of medicine in addition to the study of the heart.

An echocardiogram is recorded by placing a transducer in an interspace adjacent to the left sternal border (Fig. 8). The transducer is small and contains a piezo-electric crystal that converts electrical energy to high frequency sound waves. Thus the transducer emits sound waves into the chest that strike cardiac structures, and the sound waves (echoes) are reflected back to the chest wall. The transducer receives sound (echoes) from the cardiac structures and reconverts them to electrical energy that can then be recorded. Because the frequency of the sound waves and the speed of sound in body tissues are constant, the interval between the emission of sound and the return of sound indicates the distance into the heart that the sound wave has traveled and returned. The ultrahigh frequency sounds are reflected only from interfaces between structures of different density, as from the interface between the ventricular cavity (blood) and the ventricular septum (muscle). The amount of sound returned depends on the nature of the substances on either side of the interface. The reflecting surface must be perpendicular to the transducer, for when a surface lies tangential, the sound waves are reflected in a different direction and are not received by the transducer.

In summary, an echocardiographic transducer on the chest wall emits sound waves. As the sound waves travel into the heart, at each interface some sound is returned to the transducer, and some sound continues to the next structure where more is reflected, while some continues. In this way multiple sound waves are reflected at various distances from the surface of the chest, and these echoes can be recorded.

The ultrasonic waves can be recorded in three ways, but one of the most commonly shown is termed the M (movement) mode. In this mode, sound waves are continuously recorded over a period of time, perhaps 10 to 15 seconds. This tracing has two axes, one (vertical) representing distance from the surface of the chest and the other (horizontal) representing time. This recording allows the examiner to determine relative distances, to identify cardiac structures and their relative relationships, and to observe changes that occur with time. In the M mode the movements of cardiac structures can be recorded over several cardiac cycles. In recording the M mode the transducer does not need to be stationary but can be rotated so the direction or orientation of the transducer can be changed, allowing the examiner to record a sweep from one area of the heart to another. For example, a sweep is recorded from the aorta into the left ventricle to demonstrate the continuity between the aortic and mitral valves. Such movements of the transducer further allow identification of the relationship between cardiac structures.

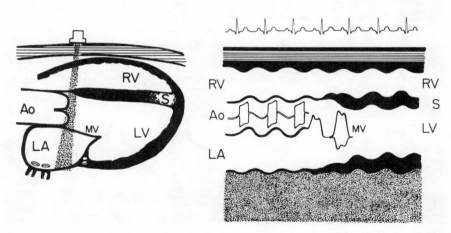

Figure 8. Diagram showing cross-section of heart and transducer beam passing through cardiac structures (left) and illustrating wave forms and chambers as viewed in echocardiographic tracing (right). These should be used to compare to Figure 9. Ao = aorta. LA = left atrium. LV = left ventricle. MV = mitral valve. RV = right ventricle. S = interventricular septum.

Echocardiography requires several components: 1) a transducer, 2) an oscilloscope to visualize the structures being recorded, and 3) a mechanism for making a permanent recording. To assist in the timing of cardiac events, an electrocardiogram is routinely recorded simultaneously with the echocardiogram. Although there are several similarities to electrocardiography, one difference is that echocardiographic technicians require a higher degree of training; they must be able to recognize wave forms and variations from normal and must have an understanding of cardiac anatomy.

The echocardiogram provides information about the heart different from that obtained from either electrocardiography or thoracic roentgenography. The right ventricular, left atrial, and left ventricular dimensions and chambers can be identified. The movements of the aortic and mitral valves are easily identified and the movements of the tricuspid and pulmonary valves are less easy to identify. Usually the diameters of both the aorta and pulmonary trunk can be determined. Furthermore, the relationships between the aorta, interventricular septum, and anterior leaflet of the mitral valve can be assessed.

In Figure 9 an echocardiogram and corresponding diagram are shown to illustrate the normal echocardiographic structures. Anteriorly, the rather

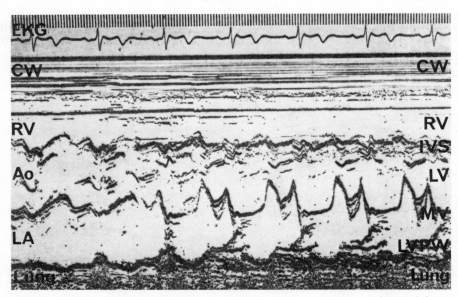

Figure 9. Echocardiogram. Continuous recording from aorta (Ao) on right into left ventricle (LV) at level of mitral valve (MV). Anteriorly is the chest wall (CW) and behind it the right ventricular cavity (RV). The interventricular septum (IVS) separates the ventricles and is continuous with anterior aortic wall. One leaflet is continuous with posterior aortic wall. EKG = electrocardiogram; LVPW = left ventricular posterior wall.

dense echoes originate from the interface between the skin and the anterior chest wall and also from the anterior wall of the right ventricle. Since this echo has several components, it is difficult to assess the thickness of the right ventricular wall. The right ventricular cavity is beneath this dense echo and is shown as a relatively echo-free space. Within the right ventricle the tricuspid valve, particularly the anterior leaflet of the tricuspid valve, can be seen. The right ventricular cavity is bounded posteriorly by the interventricular septum that is usually present in the middle of the echocardiographic tracing and is represented by bands of linear echo densities. Behind the interventricular septum lies the left ventricular cavity and then the posterior left ventricular wall. Frequently within the echoes of the left ventricular posterior wall a line appears at the endocardial surface and another distinct heavy line represents the pericardium. The thickness of the ventricular wall and the dimension of the ventricles change as the heart contracts and relaxes during the various phases of the cardiac cycle.

As the transducer is directed more cephalad within the left ventricle, the leaflets of the mitral valve can be identified. During diastole, the anterior leaflet of the mitral valve forms the letter M and the posterior leaflet simultaneously forms the letter W. During systole, the mitral valve leaflets are closed and form a linear echo near the posterior wall of the left ventricle. When the transducer is directed even more cephalad, the echo beam passes through the aorta and the left atrium. Normally the anteroposterior diameter of the left atrium equals that of the aorta. During systole, the aortic valve opens and forms a boxlike symmetrical structure within the center of the aortic diameter. During diastole, the aortic valve closes to form a narrow linear structure centrally located with the aorta. Anterior to the aorta also lie two parallel lines that represent the pulmonary trunk. Within this, the pulmonary valve movement may be visualized.

Echocardiography has several applications in the study of the child's heart. The hemodynamics may be evaluated serially by measurement of cardiac chamber size. This is particularly useful in infants with left-to-right shunts as from patent ductus arteriosus, where excess volumes are placed on the left atrium and the left ventricle. The resultant changes in the size of the left atrium and the left ventricle can be evaluated in a quantitative fashion by echocardiography. When investigating patients with cardiomegaly and no cardiac murmurs, it may help to identify pericardial effusion as an underlying cardiac condition by showing the pericardium separated from the posterior wall of the left ventricle as an echo-free space. Another application is the investigation of patients with a roentgenographic pattern of pulmonary venous obstruction by distinguishing such causes as mitral stenosis from total anomalous pulmonary venous connection. In patients with cyanotic congenital heart disease, echocardiography may show abnormalities in the interrelationship of the great vessels or overriding of the aorta. Finally, echocardiography is useful in adding additional information about patients who show unusual manifestations or unusual findings of cardiac disease.

Cardiac Catheterization

Cardiac catheterization is a widely practiced diagnostic procedure that permits the gathering of detailed information about the heart. With this technique, intracardiac pressures can be measured, oxygen saturation determined in various chambers, and contrast material injected to delineate the anatomic details of the malformation. Cardiac catheterization requires a staff of trained specialists—pediatric cardiologists, radiologists, laboratory technicians, and nurses—so that data can be obtained safely, analyzed properly, and interpreted with a high degree of accuracy.

Cardiac catheterization should be performed only after the patient has been fully evaluated by the previously described methods, and then used primarily to confirm the diagnosis and to answer specific questions frequently asked in the preparation for cardiac operation.

There are three general indications for cardiac catheterization:

1. Cardiac catheterizaton should be performed in neonates or infants with symptomatic cardiac disease who present with symptoms of congestive cardiac failure, cyanosis, or respiratory difficulties. Asymptomatic infants should not be catheterized simply because they have a cardiac murmur. The status of such infants can usually be evaluated adequately by clinical means alone; cardiac catheterization can be postponed until an age when operation is considered.

2. Asymptomatic children who are being considered for cardiac surgery should be catheterized prior to their operation. We feel that all children undergoing cardiac operation except those with patent ductus arteriosus, coarctation of the aorta, and secundum type atrial septal defect should be catheterized to confirm the diagnosis and to exclude other cardiac anomalies.

3. Many patients should be recatheterized postoperatively for evaluation of the results of cardiac operations. This is particularly important in patients who have had obstructive lesions such as aortic stenosis, pulmonary stenosis, tetralogy of Fallot, or other cardiac conditions where there are known residual abnormalities or complications from operation. In most patients with patent ductus arteriosus, atrial septal defect, and ventricular septal defect without pulmonary hypertension, cardiac catheterization is not required postoperatively unless there are residual abnormalities on clinical evaluation.

Procedure

Cardiac catheterization is performed in children in the fasting state. Sedation, with a combination of chlorpromazine, promethazine, and meperidine or morphine and phenobarbital, is frequently used. It is our policy not to sedate infants less than 1 year of age for cardiac catheterization. At some centers, general anesthesia is used.

Both the right and left sides of the heart may be catheterized either by percutaneous puncture or by operative exposure to major peripheral veins and arteries. The right side of the heart is approached either through the saphenous vein in the inguinal area or through the median basilic vein in the arm. The left side of the heart can be catheterized through two approaches: a venous catheter may be passed through the foramen ovale or atrial septal defect into the left atrium and may be manipulated further into the left ventricle, or an arterial catheter may be inserted into the brachial or femoral artery, directed into the ascending aorta, and passed in a retrograde fashion across the aortic valve into the left ventricular cavity.

Right-sided cardiac catheterization is primarily used to locate left-to-right shunts, to study pulmonary stenosis, to detect pulmonary hypertension, and to define conditions with right-to-left shunts. Left-sided cardiac catheterization is performed to evaluate anomalies of the mitral or aortic valve or to investigate left ventricular cardiomyopathies. Since arterial puncture entails more hazard than do venous studies, the echocardiogram should be considered as a less dangerous method of evaluating left heart structure and function.

Once the catheter has been inserted into the vessel, it can be advanced into the heart and with the aid of fluoroscopy can be directed into various cardiac chambers and major blood vessels. At any of these sites, pressures can be measured, blood samples can be obtained for analysis, and injection of contrast media can be made.

The catheter is connected to a pressure transducer and from this instrument pressure tracings are recorded. The pressure tracings can be analyzed and measured. The pressure values obtained are compared to normal (Table 6). Pressure data are invaluable in detecting stenotic lesions such as pulmonary stenosis, where the pressure is elevated proximal to the obstruction and is normal distally, or in identifying pulmonary hypertension.

Blood samples may be drawn from each cardiac site and analyzed for oxygen content or hemoglobin saturation. The values obtained are used principally to determine if there is a left-to-right or right-to-left shunt. Normally the oxygen saturation in each right-sided cardiac chamber is similar, but when there is an increase in the oxygen saturation in the chamber, compared to the preceding site, a left-to-right shunt has oc-

TABLE 6. NORMAL CARDIAC CATHETERIZATION VALUES

Site	Oxygen Saturation (%)	Pressure (mm Hg)
RA	70 ± 5	3-7
RV	70 ± 5	25/0
PA	70 ± 5	25/10 (mean 15)
LA	97 ± 3	5-10
LV	97 ± 3	100/0
Aorta	97 ± 3	100/70 (mean 85)

LA = left artery	RA = right artery
LV = left ventricle	RV = right ventricle
PA = pulmonary artery	

curred at that level, by definition. There are of course normal variations in oxygen content in any chamber and a slight increase may not mean a shunt. Several pairs of samples will usually resolve this point.

Normally the oxygen saturation of blood in the left atrium, the left ventricle, and the aorta should be at least 94 percent. If it is less than this level, a right-to-left shunt is present.

The pressure and oximetry data can be used to derive various measures of cardiac function. Cardiac output can be calculated using the Fick principle:

$$\text{Cardiac output (L/min)} = \frac{\text{oxygen consumption (cc/min)}}{\text{arteriovenous oxygen difference (cc/100 cc)} \times 10}$$

During cardiac catheterization, the patient's rate of oxygen consumption can be determined by analyzing a timed collection of the patient's expired air. The arteriovenous oxygen difference is obtained by analyzing blood samples drawn from the arterial side of the circulation (aorta or peripheral artery) and from the venous side of the heart (usually the pulmonary artery). The oxygen content (cc/100 cc), not percent hemoglobin saturation, is determined and used to calculate the cardiac output. Cardiac output determined by the Fick principle is widely used in analyzing catheterization data and is the standard by which other methods of cardiac output are compared.

Since many forms of congenital cardiac diseases have either a left-to-right or a right-to-left shunt, the blood flow through the lungs may differ from that through the body, even though the oxygen consumption in the latter must be equal to the oxygen picked up in the lungs. The Fick principle may still be used for such patients:

Systemic blood flow (L/min) =
(SBF)

$$\frac{\text{oxygen consumption}}{\text{arterial-mixed venous (SA-MV) oxygen difference}}$$

42

Pulmonary blood flow (L/min) =
  (PBF)

$$\frac{\text{oxygen consumption}}{\text{pulmonary vein-pulmonary arterial (PV-PA) oxygen difference}}$$

It also follows that a very useful relationship can be determined, without assuming or measuring the oxygen consumption. The pulmonary blood flow (PBF) can be expressed as a ratio of the systemic blood flow (SBF): PBF/SBF = SA-MV/PV-PA.

These formulae are based upon the fact that the difference in oxygen must be measured across the vascular system in question: systemic vascular system—arterial (aorta or systemic artery) and venous (from a right-sided chamber proximal to a shunt); and pulmonary vascular system—pulmonary vein (blood coming from the lungs) and the pulmonary artery (blood entering the lungs).

If there is a shunt in either direction, the arteriovenous oxygen differences are not equal across the two vascular systems. In a left-to-right shunt, pulmonary blood flow exceeds systemic blood flow, and the arteriovenous oxygen difference across the lung is less than across the systemic circuit. In a pure right-to-left shunt, the opposite is true; the pulmonary blood flow is less than the systemic flow, and the arteriovenous oxygen differences are greater across the lung and are higher than across the systemic circuit.

From the data obtained at catheterization, systemic and pulmonary vascular resistances can be calculated from the equation

$$R = \frac{P}{F}$$

where
R = resistance, P = mean arterial pressure, F = cardiac output.

Therefore:

$$\text{Systemic vascular resistance} = \frac{\text{mean aortic pressure (mm Hg)}}{\text{systemic blood flow (L/min/m}^2)}$$
(mm Hg/L/min/m^2)

Pulmonary vascular resistance =
  (mm Hg/L/min/m^2)

$$\frac{\text{mean pulmonary arterial pressure (mm Hg)}}{\text{pulmonary blood flow (L/min/m}^2)}$$

Complications of Cardiac Catheterization

As with any procedure, cardiac catheterization may be associated with complications, including death. In any patient, the benefits from cardiac catheterization must clearly outweigh the risks.

43

Death may occur during or immediately after cardiac catheterization of infants and children, although this is extremely uncommon (0.1 percent) in children beyond 1 year of age. The risk is higher in infants, particularly neonates (3 percent). These patients are often critically ill and require the procedure to identify the cardiac condition so that a lifesaving procedure can be performed. All children undergoing cardiac catheterization should be carefully monitored. In neonates, temperature, acid-base balance, blood pressure, pulse, and respiratory and blood loss must be followed closely.

During most cardiac catheterizations, arrhythmias of some type occur, but these usually are transient and rarely compromise the patient unless he is in congestive cardiac failure or is intensely cyanotic.

Angiocardiography

At the time of catheterization, contrast material can be injected through the catheter into the cardiac chambers and serial x-ray pictures can be obtained in rapid succession, or movies can be made (cine technique), often in two projections simultaneously. An excellent view of the cardiac anatomy is obtained so that the details of the cardiac chambers, valves, and great vessels are delineated. The technique is particularly useful in showing the site and the form of a right-to-left shunt. Stenotic lesions of the aorta and the pulmonary valves are outlined by these methods, but the severity of the lesion can be judged only by catheterization data.

Aortography

Aortography is useful in the diagnosis of lesions of the aortic arch such as coarctation of the aorta or patent ductus arteriosus. Contrast material is injected either through a catheter placed in the ascending aorta or in a retrograde fashion from the brachial artery. By opacification of the aortic arch, one can define the aorta and any abnormalities of its structure. In infants without a left-to-right shunt, satisfactory details may be obtained by injecting into the pulmonary artery and filming as the contrast passes through the left side of the heart.

3

SPECIFIC CONGENITAL
CARDIAC MALFORMATIONS

Congenital cardiac malformations may be classified in various ways. A clinically useful classification is based on two clinical features: the presence or absence of cyanosis and the type of pulmonary vascularity, increased, normal, or diminished. Six subgroups of malformations are therefore possible, and within each subgroup the malformations result in similar hemodynamic alterations. The thirteen cardiac malformations classified in Table 7 represent the major congenital cardiac defects and are present in 80 percent of children with congenital cardiac disease. Certain exceptions to this classification occur in infancy, and will be discussed later.

Before we proceed with the presentation of detailed information concerning the individual cardiac malformations, several hemodynamic principles will be discussed.

HEMODYNAMIC PRINCIPLES

The first principle concerns conditions with a communication between the great vessels or between the ventricles, examples of these being patent ductus arteriosus and ventricular septal defect, respectively. The direction and magnitude of flow through such a communication is dependent either on the size of the communication or on the relative resistances to systemic and pulmonary blood flow. In defects or communications smaller than the diameter of the aortic root, the systolic pressure difference across the communication is the major determining factor governing the direction and magnitude of the blood flow through the communication. Because the aortic and left ventricular systolic pressures are higher than the pulmonary

TABLE 7. CLASSIFICATION OF MAJOR CARDIAC MALFORMATIONS

Pulmonary Vascularity	Acyanotic	Cyanotic (Right-to-Left Shunt)
Increased	*Left-to-right shunts* **Ventricular septal defect** **Patent ductus arteriosus** **Endocardial cushion defect** **Atrial septal defect**	*Admixture lesions* **Complete transposition of great vessels** **Total anomalous pulmonary venous connection** **Truncus arteriosus**
Normal	*Obstructive lesions* **Aortic stenosis** **Pulmonary stenosis** **Coarctation of aorta** *Cardiomyopathy*	None
Decreased	None	*Obstruction to pulmonary blood flow + defect* **Tetralogy of Fallot** **Tricuspid atresia** **Ebstein's malformation of tricuspid valve**

arterial and right ventricular pressures, respectively, the shunt in these small-sized communications is from the aorta to the pulmonary artery or from the left ventricle to the right ventricle.

When the defect or communication approaches or exceeds the diameter of the aortic root, the systolic pressures in the ventricles and great vessels are equal, those on the right side of the heart being elevated to systemic levels.

In patients with large communications at the ventricular or great vessel level, the direction and magnitude of the shunt are dependent upon the relative pulmonary and systemic vascular resistances. These resistances in turn are directly related to the caliber and number of pulmonary and systemic arterioles. Normally systemic vascular resistance rises slowly with age, while the pulmonary vascular resistance shows a sharp fall in the neonatal and infancy period. This fall in pulmonary vascular resistance is partially related to regression of the thick-walled pulmonary arterioles of the fetal period to the adult pattern of pulmonary arterioles which show a wide lumen. Pulmonary vascular resistance falls in all infants following birth, but it is in infants with a large communication that the fall in pulmonary vascular resistance has a profound effect.

In a large communication the systolic pressure of the pulmonary artery (P) remains constant and is determined largely by the systemic arterial pressure. Therefore, according to the formula $P = R \times F$, as the pulmonary vascular resistance (R) falls in infancy, pulmonary blood flow (F) increases. If some factor such as the development of pulmonary vascular disease should increase pulmonary vascular resistance, the pulmonary blood flow would decrease, while the pulmonary arterial pressure remains constant.

The second hemodynamic principle governs shunts that occur at the atrial level. Most atrial communications that lead to signs and symptoms are large, thus the atrial pressures are equal. Therefore, pressure differences are not the primary determinate of blood flow through the atrial communication. The direction and magnitude are determined rather by the relative compliances of the atria and the ventricles. In contrast to the shunts at the ventricular or great vessel level, which are influenced by the relative resistances of the pulmonary and systemic beds and therefore systolic events, shunts at the atrial level are governed by factors influencing ventricular filling.

Compliance is volume change per unit pressure change. Therefore for any given pressure, the more compliant the ventricle the greater the volume it can receive. Ventricular compliance is dependent upon the thickness of the ventricular wall and factors such as fibrosis that alters the stiffness of the ventricle. Usually, the thinner the ventricular wall, the more compliant the ventricle. Normally the left ventricle is thicker-walled and less compliant than the thin-walled right ventricle. This difference in compliance favors blood flow from the left atrium to the right atrium in patients with atrial communication. In addition, this direction of blood flow is favored because the right atrium is also more compliant than the left atrium since the vena cava adds to the reservoir of the right atrium.

The direction and volume of shunt can be altered by changes in the degree of thickness of the ventricular walls or by factors such as myocardial fibrosis.

Right ventricular compliance increases during infancy, as a result of the changes in pulmonary vascular resistance. During fetal life, the right ventricle develops systemic levels of pressure, since it ejects a large portion of its output across the ductus arteriosus into the aorta. Therefore the right ventricle is thick-walled and, at birth, weighs twice as much as the left ventricle. Since ventricular compliance is affected by the thickness of the ventricular wall, at birth the right ventricle is relatively less compliant.

Following birth, the pulmonary vascular resistance decreases, and right ventricular systolic pressure falls to a normal level (25 mm Hg). As a consequence, the right ventricular wall thins, and by 1 month the left ventricular weight exceeds that of the right ventricle. The thinning of the wall is associated with an increase in right ventricular compliance. While this sequence occurs in every neonate, in those with an atrial septal defect, as right ventricular compliance increases, so does the volume of left-to-right shunt.

The third hemodynamic principle concerns cardiac conditions with obstruction to blood flow. The primary response to obstruction is hypertrophy, not dilatation. Pressure increases in the chamber proximal to the obstruction, leading to hypertrophy of that chamber. In children the pressure is usually maintained distal to the obstruction, since the cardiac output is also usually maintained. Many of the signs and symptoms of patients with obstruction are related to the pressure elevation proximal to the obstruction.

The fourth principle governs conditions with valvular insufficiency. The chamber on either side of the insufficient valve is enlarged. The volume of blood in each chamber is larger than normal because the chambers are handling not only the normal cardiac output but the regurgitant volume also. The response of the increased volume is usually ventricular enlargement, in contrast to conditions with obstruction, where the response is hypertrophy. The major signs and symptoms of these patients are related to enlargement of the chambers.

The term *pulmonary hypertension* must also be defined before considering specific cardiac malformations. Pulmonary hypertension indicates an elevation of pulmonary arterial pressure. As indicated by the equation $P = R \times F$, pressure (in this case pulmonary arterial pressure) equals the resistance (R) to blood flow through the lungs and the volume of pulmonary blood flow (F). Therefore, for any given level of pressure, various combinations of pressure and blood flow may be present.

Pulmonary arterial pressure may be elevated primarily from increased pulmonary blood flow secondary to a left-to-right shunt, as in a large ventricular septal defect or patent ductus arteriosus.

Pulmonary arterial pressure may also be elevated secondary to elevated resistance to blood flow through the lungs. The elevated resistance may occur at either of two sites in the pulmonary circulation: at a precapillary site (usually the pulmonary arterioles) or at a postcapillary site (such as the pulmonary veins, the left atrium, or the mitral valve).

At a precapillary site, pulmonary hypertension results from narrowing of the pulmonary arterioles. At birth the pulmonary arterioles show a thick medial coat and a narrow lumen, and the pulmonary resistance is elevated. With time, as indicated previously, the media of the arteriole thins and the lumen opens, so the pulmonary resistance falls. The arterioles of infants are responsive to various influences, such as oxygen and acidosis. With hypoxia they may contract further and with administration of oxygen they may widen. Such responsiveness may present longer in infants with cardiac malformation associated with increased pulmonary blood flow and elevated pressures.

Pulmonary resistance may also be elevated because of acquired lesions in the pulmonary arterioles. In patients with large pulmonary blood flow and elevated pulmonary arterial pressure, pulmonary vascular disease develops and medial thickening and intimal proliferation occur. These changes develop at a variable rate. Such changes influence the clinical findings of patients and the operative results and mortality. If these fixed

48

changes are present, the operative risk is high, and the pulmonary resistance remains elevated following operation.

Pulmonary arterial pressure may also be elevated by malformations that cause obstruction to blood flow beyond the pulmonary capillary (such as in the pulmonary veins, the left atrium, or across the mitral valve). The classic example is mitral stenosis, in which the pulmonary arterial pressure is passively elevated because of elevation of the left atrium and subsequent elevation of pulmonary venous and capillary pressures. In addition some patients with obstruction at this level show reflex pulmonary arteriole vasoconstriction, further elevating the pulmonary arterial pressure.

These two sites leading to elevation of pulmonary arterial pressure can usually be distinguished clinically, although both show a loud P_2 and right ventricular hypertrophy, reflecting the pulmonary hypertension. In the postcapillary form, usually there are signs of pulmonary venous hypertension, such as pulmonary edema and Kerley B lines. Cardiac catheterization also allows separation by measurement of the pulmonary wedge pressure. Wedge pressure is obtained by advancing the catheter as far into the pulmonary artery as possible. At this site the pulmonary artery is occluded so the pressure recorded reflects the pressure in the vascular bed beyond the catheter. The pressure recording is of the pulmonary capillary pressure that reflects pulmonary venous pressure. In pulmonary hypertension secondary to a postcapillary obstruction, the wedge pressure is elevated; whereas in the precapillary origin, the wedge pressure is normal.

During the evaluation of patients with cardiac anomalies, a variety of information is obtained clinically. The signs, symptoms, and laboratory data can conveniently be divided into three categories to permit a better understanding of the physiologic significance of the findings and of the patient's condition. In the first category are findings indicating the cardiac diagnosis; in the second, the severity of the condition; and in the third, features that may suggest an etiology.

In the first category belong those findings, usually auscultatory, that are related directly to the abnormality. These are usually related to turbulent flow through the defect or abnormality; examples are the continuous murmur of a patent ductus arteriosus and the aortic ejection murmur of aortic stenosis. The findings in this category indicate the cardiac diagnosis.

In the second category are findings that reflect the effect of the malformation upon the circulation, used to assess the severity of the malformation. Often symptoms, electrocardiographic and roentgenographic findings, and certain auscultatory findings belong in this category.

Since several malformations may have similar effects upon the circulation, as for example ventricular septal defect and patent ductus arteriosus in which each places increased volume loads on the left atrium and left ventricle, similar secondary features may be found in each. In this example the clinical and laboratory features indicating enlargement of these chambers will be clinically evident, and the degree of enlargement roughly paralleled by the magnitude of symptoms and laboratory changes. In either of these conditions, for example, if the communication is sufficiently large, congestive cardiac failure, apical diastolic murmur, left ventricular hypertrophy, and cardiomegaly are found.

ACYANOSIS AND INCREASED PULMONARY BLOOD FLOW (LEFT-TO-RIGHT SHUNT)

The combination of increased pulmonary vascular markings and absence of cyanosis indicates the presence of a cardiac defect that permits the passage of blood from a left-sided cardiac chamber to a right-sided cardiac chamber. Four cardiac defects account for most instances of left-to-right shunt: 1) ventricular septal defect; 2) patent ductus arteriosus; 3) atrial septal defect of the ostium secundum type; and 4) endocardial cushion defect. In the first two conditions, the direction and magnitude of the shunt are governed by factors influencing shunts at either the ventricular level or the great vessel level; namely, relative resistances if the defect is large and relative pressures if the communication is small. In most cases, the resistances and pressures on the right side of the heart and the pulmonary arterial system are less than on the left side of the heart, and a left-to-right shunt occurs.

In atrial septal defect and endocardial cushion defect, since the shunt occurs at the atrial level, ventricular compliances influence the shunt. Since the right ventricle normally is more compliant than the left, a left-to-right shunt occurs in these patients also.

In certain circumstances, the shunt in these malformations may become right to left; this state will be discussed more fully later.

The clinical and laboratory findings of any given condition may vary considerably with the volume of pulmonary blood flow, the status of pulmonary vasculature, and the presence of coexistent cardiac anomalies.

Although many patients with these malformations are asymptomatic, symptoms of poor growth and congestive cardiac failure occur in patients with greatly increased blood flow, as in ventricular septal defect and patent ductus arteriosus. There is a tendency for frequent respiratory infections and episodes of pneumonia.

In this section, the factors governing flow through ventricular septal defects and through atrial septal defects will be discussed in greater detail. This information should be carefully studied and mastered, for it can be applied in subsequent sections for understanding more complex anomalies with communication between the two sides of circulation.

Ventricular Septal Defect

Ventricular septal defect (Fig. 10) is the most frequently occurring congenital cardiac anomaly, accounting for nearly one fourth of all cases. A ventricular septal defect is a component of the cardiac malformation in about one half of all patients with congenital cardiac anomalies.

Isolated ventricular septal defects are most frequently located in the area of the membranous portion of the ventricular septum, but may occasionally be located above the crista supraventricularis or in the muscular portion of the septum. The location of the defect, while not nearly as important as the size of the defect in determining the clinical manifestation, does influence the operative approach.

As a result of the defect, shunting of blood can occur between the ventricles. When the size of the defect approaches the size of the aortic annulus, flow is governed by the relative pulmonary and systemic vascular resistances. When the defect is smaller, the blood flows from the left to the right ventricle because of the higher systolic pressure in the left ventricle. As there are two physiologic mechanisms influencing the shunt in ventricular septal defect, the clinical findings, natural history, and operative considerations for these two sized defects will be considered separately.

LARGE VENTRICULAR SEPTAL DEFECT

In patients whose ventricular septal defect approaches the size of the aorta, the resistance to outflow from the heart is determined primarily by the caliber of the arterioles of the respective vascular beds. Since the systemic arterioles have a thick muscular coat and narrow lumen and the pulmonary arterioles have a thin coat and wide lumen, the systemic resistance is greater than the pulmonary resistance. In a normal individual, that is, someone without a left-to-right shunt, this is reflected by systemic arterial pressure in the range of 110/70 mm Hg and by pulmonary arterial pressure of 25/10 mm Hg.

Since the flow through a larger defect is governed by resistances, any condition that increases resistance to left ventricular outflow, such as coarctation of the aorta or aortic stenosis, increases the magnitude of the left-to-right shunt; whereas any abnormality that obstructs right ventricular outflow, such as coexistent pulmonary stenosis, as in tetralogy of Fallot or pulmonary arteriolar disease, decreases the magnitude of the left-to-right shunt. Indeed, if the resistance to right ventricular outflow is greater than the resistance to left ventricular outflow, the shunt may be in a right-to-left direction.

Prior to and at birth the pulmonary vascular resistance is elevated and is greater than the systemic vascular resistance. In the newborn, the pulmonary arterioles are thick-walled and resemble histologically sys-

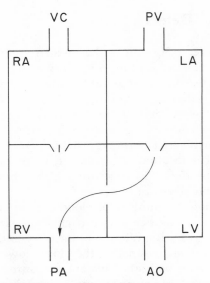

Figure 10. Central circulation in isolated ventricular septal defect. Ao = aorta. LA = left atrium. LV = left ventricle. PA = pulmonary artery. PV = pulmonary vein. RA = right atrium. RV = right ventricle. VC = vena cava.

temic arterioles. The elevation of pulmonary vascular resistance prior to birth is supported by observations of the fetal circulation, in which the right ventricular output enters the pulmonary artery; the major portion flows into the aorta through the ductus arteriosus and only a small portion enters the lungs. The proportions of flow to each vascular bed depend on the relative resistances. This feature of the neonatal circulation indicates the elevation of pulmonary vascular resistance in relation to systemic vascular resistance.

Following birth, the pulmonary arterioles change. The media becomes thinner and the lumen becomes wider (Fig. 11). Thus the pulmonary vascular resistance falls, reaching nearly adult levels by the time the child is about 8 weeks of age. Although this sequence occurs in every individual, this decrease in pulmonary vascular resistance has profound effects on patients with ventricular septal defect. In patients with a large ventricular septal defect, the medial layer does not undergo regression either as quickly as or to the extent of that of normal individuals, so that at any age the pulmonary vascular resistance is higher than normal, yet lower than the systemic resistance.

In patients with a large isolated ventricular septal defect, the systolic pressure in both ventricles and great vessels is the same, with the right-sided pressures being elevated to equal those normally present on the left side of the heart. Systolic pressure in the aorta is regulated at a constant level by baroreceptors. Therefore, in large ventricular septal defects, the pulmonary artery pressure (P) is relatively fixed. According to $P = R \times F$, as the pulmonary vascular resistance (R) falls, the volume of pulmonary blood flow (F) increases. This is in contrast to the events occurring in an infant without a shunt, where pulmonary blood flow (F) is constant; therefore, according to $P = R \times F$, as pulmonary resistance (R) falls following birth, so does the pulmonary arterial pressure (P).

Among patients with a large ventricular septal defect, at whatever level of pulmonary arterial pressure, as the pulmonary resistance falls consequent to the maturation of the pulmonary vessels, the volume of pulmonary blood flow increases. At birth there may be little flow across the defect, but as the child grows the flow increases.

Large ventricular septal defects place two major hemodynamic loads upon the ventricles: increased pressure load on the right ventricle and increased volume load on the left ventricle.

In large defects the right ventricle develops a level of systolic pressure equal to that of the left ventricle. The right ventricular work load is proportional to the level of pulmonary arterial pressure ($P = R \times F$). Pulmonary arterial hypertension can result either from increased pulmonary arterial resistance or from increased pulmonary blood flow. Regardless of the origin of pulmonary hypertension, the right ventricle is thick-walled, but its state has really not changed from fetal life when it was also developing high levels of pressure. Since the pressure remained elevated postnatally, the normal evolution of the right ventricle to a thin-walled, crescent-shaped chamber does not occur. The right ventricle can tolerate and maintain these levels of pressure without the development of cardiac failure.

In ventricular septal defect and left-to-right shunt, there is volume overload of the left ventricle because this chamber must not only maintain the systemic blood flow but must eject blood through the ventricular septal defect into the lungs. When the ventricles contract, the flow from the left ventricle through the ventricular septal defect is directed almost entirely into the pulmonary artery, so that the right ventricle has little excess volume load. The augmented pulmonary blood flow returns through the left atrium to the left ventricle. To accommodate the increased pulmonary venous return, the left ventricle dilates (Fig. 12). As dilatation occurs, the radius and circumference of the left ventricle increase and the myocardial fibers lengthen. Both the Laplace and Starling laws describe this relationship. The Laplace relationship states that in a cylindrical object, as the radius increases, the tension (T) in the wall must also increase to maintain pressure ($T = P \times R$). Therefore, as the left ventricle dilates and increases its radius, it must develop increased wall tension to maintain ventricular pressure. If the left ventricle becomes greatly dilated, the myocardium cannot develop sufficient tension to maintain its pressure volume rela-

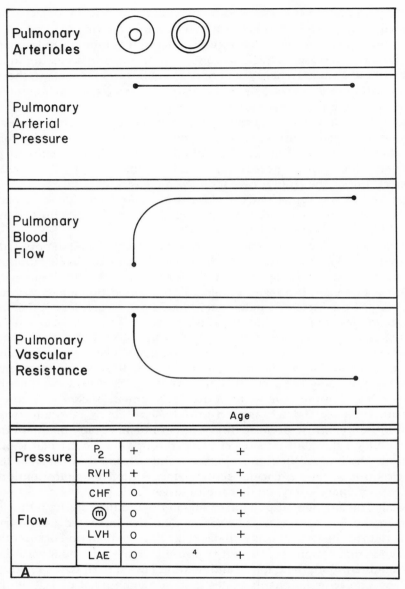

Pulmonary Arterioles				
Pulmonary Arterial Pressure				
Pulmonary Blood Flow				
Pulmonary Vascular Resistance				
		Age		

Pressure	P₂	+		+
	RVH	+		+
Flow	CHF	0		+
	ⓜ	0		+
	LVH	0		+
	LAE	0	4	+

A

Figure 11. A. Changes in pulmonary arterial pressure, pulmonary blood flow, and pulmonary vascular resistance in an infant with a large ventricular septal defect. Correlation with major clinical findings reflecting pulmonary arterial pressure and pulmonary blood flow. CHF = congestive heart failure. LAE = left atrial enlargement. LVH = left ventricular hypertrophy. M = murmur. P_2 = pulmonary component of second heart sound. RVH = right ventricular hypertrophy. B. Changes in pulmonary arterial pressure, pulmonary blood flow, and pulmonary vascular resistances in a normal infant.

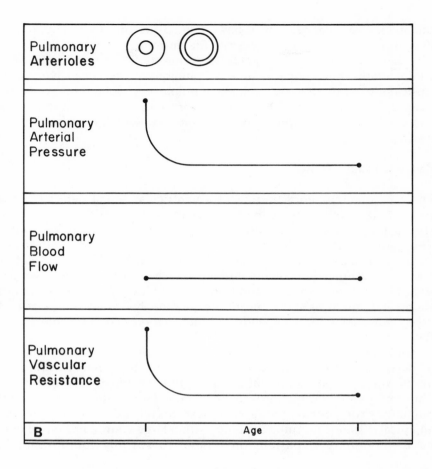

tionship, and congestive cardiac failure occurs. Starling's law states that as myocardial fiber is stretched, cardiac function increases to a point beyond which function falls.

The signs and symptoms of a large ventricular septal defect vary with the relative vascular resistances and the volume of pulmonary blood flow. In evaluating a patient with a large ventricular septal defect, attention should be directed diagnostically for information that permits definition of pulmonary blood flow (F) and pulmonary artery pressure (P) so that an estimate of pulmonary vascular resistance (R) can be obtained.

History

In many patients with a large ventricular septal defect, the murmur may not be heard until the first postnatal visit to the physician. By that age the pulmonary vascular resistance has fallen sufficiently that enough blood flows through the defect to generate the murmur.

Patients with a larger-sized defect develop congestive cardiac failure by 2 to 3 months of age. By this time the pulmonary arterioles have matured sufficiently to permit a large volume of pulmonary blood flow. As a consequence, left ventricular dilatation develops and results in cardiac failure and its associated symptoms of tachypnea, slow weight gain, and poor feeding.

Physical Examination

The classic auscultatory finding of a ventricular septal defect is a loud pansystolic murmur heard best in the third and fourth left intercostal spaces. Usually associated with a thrill, the murmur is widely transmitted. The murmur begins with the first heart sound and includes the isovolumetric contraction period of the cardiac cycle. Since the ventricles are in communication, blood shunts from the left to the right ventricle from the onset of systole. The murmur usually lasts until the second heart sound. The loudness of the murmur is not directly related to the size of the defect, for the loudness depends on other factors such as volume of blood flow through the defect.

In addition to recognizing the murmur and diagnosing ventricular septal defect, the clinician must also describe other auscultatory features that define the pulmonary arterial pressure and the pulmonary blood flow. This important information can be obtained from the intensity of the pulmonary component of the second heart sound and from the presence of an apical diastolic murmur. Patients with a large ventricular septal defect have pulmonary hypertension related to various combinations of

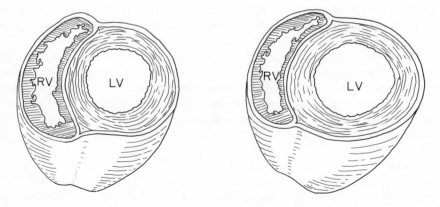

Figure 12. Cross-section through ventricles. Normal contour shown on left. Dilated left ventricle in ventricular septal defect (right). LV = left ventricle. RV = right ventricle.

pulmonary blood flow and increased pulmonary vascular resistance. Regardless of the cause, pulmonary hypertension is indicated by an increased intensity of the pulmonary component of the second heart sound. The louder the pulmonary component, the higher the pulmonary arterial pressure.

In patients with a large ventricular septal defect and a large volume of pulmonary blood flow, the volume of pulmonary venous blood crossing the mitral valve into the left ventricle during diastole is greatly increased. When the volume of blood flow across the mitral valve exceeds twice normal, a diastolic inflow murmur is heard. The murmur occurs in mid-diastole, often following a third heart sound. It is low pitched and heard best at the cardiac apex. The loudness roughly parallels the volume of pulmonary blood flow.

By combining the knowledge of the intensity of the second heart sound and the presence or absence of the diastolic murmur, valuable knowledge of the status of the pulmonary vascular bed is obtained. An increased pulmonary component of the second heart sound indicates pulmonary hypertension, whether caused by increased pulmonary blood flow or by increased pulmonary vascular resistance. In the presence of a diastolic murmur, the loud pulmonic valve closure is primarily related to increased pulmonary flow. The absence of a mitral murmur indicates that the pulmonary hypertension is secondary to increased pulmonary vascular resistance.

Clinical evidence of cardiomegaly may be present in those patients with increased pulmonary blood flow either by the finding of a cardiac apex that is displaced laterally and inferiorly, or by a precordial bulge. The findings of cardiomegaly and hepatomegaly support the diagnosis of congestive cardiac failure. In addition, tachypnea, tachycardia, and dyspnea in the infant suggest congestive cardiac failure.

Electrocardiographic Features

The electrocardiogram reflects the types of hemodynamic load placed upon the ventricles: left ventricular volume overload related to increased pulmonary blood flow, and right ventricular pressure overload related to pulmonary hypertension. The electrocardiogram varies, depending upon the hemodynamics, but findings of left ventricular hypertrophy reflect the volume of pulmonary blood flow, and findings of right ventricular hypertrophy indicate the level of right ventricular systolic pressure paralleling the pulmonary arterial pressure. In patients with a large volume of pulmonary blood flow and pulmonary hypertension related to that flow, biventricular (combined) hypertrophy is present (Fig. 13). A pattern of isolated right ventricular hypertrophy and right axis deviation occurs in patients with pulmonary hypertension related to increased pulmonary vascular resistance of any cause. The increased pulmonary vascular resistance limits pulmonary blood flow, and therefore a pattern of left ventricular hypertrophy is not present.

Roentgenographic Features

The pulmonary vasculature appears normal at birth but increases soon thereafter. The roentgenographic appearance of the heart varies according to the magnitude of the shunt and the level of pulmonary arterial pressure. The size ranges from normal to markedly enlarged; it varies directly with the magnitude of the shunt. The cardiac enlargement results from enlargement of both the left atrium and the left ventricle from the increased flow. The left atrium is a particularly valuable indicator of pulmonary blood flow because this chamber can be easily assessed roentgenographically. The right ventricular hypertrophy in itself does not contribute to cardiac enlargement. The pulmonary artery can be enlarged because of the volume of pulmonary blood flow or pulmonary hypertension.

There is no characteristic contour of the heart in ventricular septal defect.

Summary of Clinical Findings

The primary finding of ventricular septal defect is a pansystolic murmur along the left sternal border.

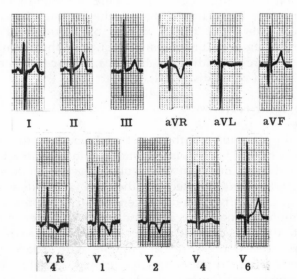

Figure 13. Electrocardiogram in ventricular septal defect. Normal QRS axis and P waves. Pattern of biventricular hypertrophy. Tall R wave in leads V_4R and V_1 indicates right ventricular hypertrophy. Deep Q wave and tall R wave in lead V_6 indicate volume overload of left ventricle.

58

The secondary features of ventricular septal defect reflect the components of the equation $P = R \times F$. The pulmonary arterial pressure (P) is indicated by the loudness of the pulmonary component of the second heart sound and by the degree of right ventricular hypertrophy on the electrocardiogram. Pulmonary blood flow (F) is indicated by a history of congestive cardiac failure, an apical diastolic murmur, left ventricular hypertrophy on the electrocardiogram, cardiomegaly, and left atrial enlargement on thoracic roentgenogram.

The changes with age of the secondary features are shown in Figure 11.

Natural History

Patients with an uncorrected large ventricular septal defect may follow one of three courses.

1. *Pulmonary vascular disease may develop.* The initiating factors causing the development of medial hypertrophy and later intimal proliferation are unknown, but they are probably related principally to the fact that the arterioles are being submitted to high levels of pressure and, to a lesser degree, to elevated blood flow. The anatomic changes can develop in pulmonary arterioles of children as young as 1 year. The initial changes of medial hypertrophy are in large part reversible if the ventricular septal defect is corrected, but the intimal changes are permanent. The pathologic changes of the pulmonary arterioles are usually progressive unless the course is interrupted by operation.

The result of these anatomic changes is progressive elevation of pulmonary vascular resistance (Fig. 14). The pulmonary arterial pressure does not increase, but rather stays constant because the ventricles are in free communication. Therefore, the volume of pulmonary blood flow decreases.

Eventually the pulmonary vascular resistance may become greater than systemic vascular resistance, at which time the shunt becomes right to left through the defect, and cyanosis develops.

The progressive rise in pulmonary vascular resistance can be followed clinically by observing the changes in the secondary features of ventricular septal defect. Those features reflecting elevated arterial pressure, right ventricular hypertrophy, and loudness of the pulmonary component remain constant; while those reflecting pulmonary blood flow change (Fig. 14).

Thus these clinical findings reflecting the excessive flow through the left side of the heart gradually disappear. Congestive cardiac failure lessens, the diastolic murmur fades, the electrocardiogram no longer shows the left ventricular hypertrophy, and the cardiac size is reduced on thoracic roentgenogram. The heart size is normal because the total volume of blood is normal. The right ventricle is hypertrophied, but this does not cause

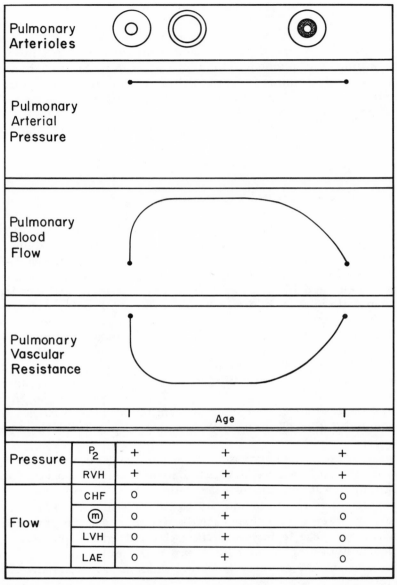

Figure 14. Changes in pulmonary arterial pressure, pulmonary blood flow, and pulmonary vascular resistances in a patient with a large ventricular septal defect who develops pulmonary vascular disease. Correlation with major clinical findings reflecting pulmonary arterial pressure and pulmonary blood flow. CHF = congestive heart failure. LAE = left atrial enlargement. LVH = left ventricular hypertrophy. M = murmur. P_2 = pulmonary component of second heart sound. RVH = right ventricular hypertrophy.

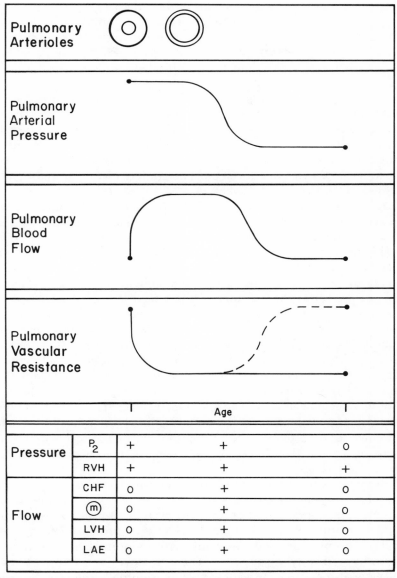

Figure 15. Changes in pulmonary arterial pressure, pulmonary blood flow, and pulmonary vascular resistances in a patient with a large ventricular septal defect who develops infundibular pulmonary stenosis. Correlation with major clinical findings reflecting pulmonary arterial pressure and pulmonary blood flow. Interrupted line indicates resistance imposed by infundibular stenosis. CHF = congestive heart failure. LAE = left atrial enlargement. LVH = left ventricular hypertrophy. M = murmur. P_2 = pulmonary component of second heart sound. RVH = right ventricular hypertrophy.

enlargement. For many patients with cardiac disease, the disappearance of congestive cardiac failure and the presence of a normal heart size is considered favorable, but in this instance these changes are ominous.

2. *Infundibular pulmonary stenosis may develop.* In certain patients with a large ventricular septal defect, infundibular stenosis may develop and progressively narrow the right ventricular outflow area. In such patients, this stenotic area represents a major resistance to outflow into the lungs, and the pulmonary vascular resistance is often normal (Fig. 15). The shunt in these patients is influenced by the relationship between the systemic vascular resistance and the resistance imposed by the infundibular stenosis. Eventually the latter may exceed the former so the shunt becomes right to left and cyanosis develops. The clinical picture of these patients then resembles tetralogy of Fallot.

In these patients, the loudness of the pulmonary component becomes normal or reduced and delayed, but right ventricular hypertrophy persists because the right ventricle is still developing systemic levels of pressure. The features related to pulmonary blood flow—congestive cardiac failure, apical diastolic murmur, left ventricular hypertrophy on the electrocardiogram, cardiomegaly, and left atrial enlargement on thoracic roentgenogram—disappear as the pulmonary blood flow is reduced.

Regardless of whether the resistance to pulmonary blood flow resides in the infundibulum or the pulmonary arterioles, the hemodynamic effects are similar, although the prognosis is entirely dissimilar.

3. *The ventricular septal defect may undergo spontaneous closure.* The exact incidence of spontaneous closure is unknown, but perhaps up to 5 percent of large ventricular septal defects undergo spontaneous closure, and others become smaller. The spontaneous closure occurs by two basic mechanisms: by adherence of the septal leaflet of the tricuspid valve to the ventricular septum, thereby occluding the ventricular septal defect, or by closure of a muscular defect by ingrowth of myocardium and finally fibrous proliferation.

Most instances of spontaneous closure occur by 3 years of age, when the pulmonary vascular resistance is still near normal levels. As the closure of the ventricular septal defect occurs, the systolic murmur softens and the secondary features reflecting pulmonary arterial pressure become normal (Fig. 16). The pulmonary component becomes normal and the right ventricular hypertrophy disappears. Those features reflecting pulmonary blood flow also gradually disappear. Thus eventually the systolic murmur disappears, and there are no residual cardiac abnormalities, although the heart may remain large for some months.

Cardiac Catheterization

Cardiac catheterization is indicated in all patients with a large ventricular septal defect and congestive cardiac failure. The purposes of the procedure are to define the hemodynamics, identify coexistent cardiac anomalies, and localize the site of the ventricular septal defect.

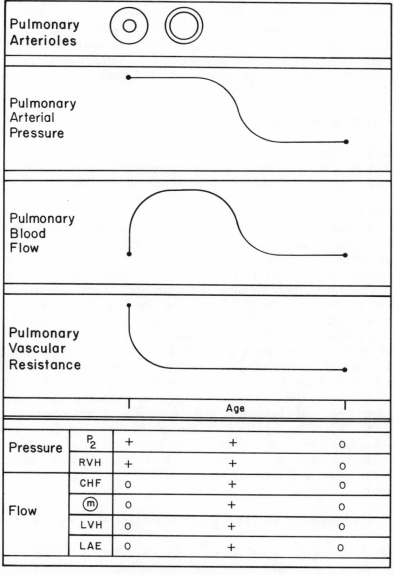

Figure 16. Changes in pulmonary arterial pressure, pulmonary blood flow, and pulmonary vascular resistances in a patient with a large ventricular septal defect which undergoes spontaneous closure. Correlation with major clinical findings reflecting pulmonary arterial pressure and pulmonary blood flow. CHF = congestive heart failure. LAE = left atrial enlargement. LVH = left ventricular hypertrophy. M = murmur. P_2 = pulmonary component of second heart sound. RVH = right ventricular hypertrophy.

A large increase in oxygen saturation is found at the right ventricular level. The pulmonary arterial and right ventricular systolic pressures are identical to those in the aorta and the left ventricle. As the pulmonary vascular resistance increases, the increase in oxygen saturation decreases and the pulmonary arterial pressure remains the same.

In these infants, ventriculography is indicated to locate the position of the ventricular septal defect because the location influences operative repair. Aortography should also be performed to exclude a coexistent patent ductus arteriosus, which may be a silent partner.

Operative Considerations

Patients with large ventricular septal defect and congestive cardiac failure should be treated with digitalis and other measures, such as diuretics and salt restriction. Although these measures improve the clinical status, many patients frequently show persistent findings of cardiac failure, so that operative treatment is indicated.

There are two operative procedures available: banding of the pulmonary artery and corrective operations. Banding of the pulmonary artery has previously been the preferred treatment for infants with ventricular septal defect and congestive cardiac failure, but at most centers corrective operations are now preferred. Banding of the pulmonary artery causes an increase in the resistance to blood flow into the lungs, and therefore the volume of blood flow returning to the left side of the heart is reduced. As a result the congestive cardiac failure improves.

Banding of the pulmonary artery provides palliation, but a second operation is required to correct the cardiac condition and to remove the band. Abnormalities of the pulmonary artery or the pulmonary valve can develop secondary to the band, may persist after removal of the band, and may present residual obstruction to the pulmonary blood flow.

Corrective operation for closure of the ventricular septal defect is indicated in infancy for those patients with persistent cardiac failure and pulmonary hypertension. The operative risk for this procedure in infants is about 10 percent. The long-term results of the procedure are yet to be evaluated.

SMALL OR MEDIUM VENTRICULAR SEPTAL DEFECTS

The size of ventricular septal defects varies considerably. In the previous section, those defects whose diameter approached the size of the aortic annulus were discussed. In this section, smaller ventricular septal defects are discussed.

The direction and magnitude of blood flow in small or medium ventricular septal defects are dependent upon the size of the defect and the pressure difference between the left ventricle and the right ventricle. The pulmonary arterial pressures are lower than the systemic pressures because the defect limits the transmission of left ventricular systolic pressure to the right side of the heart. While in large ventricular septal defects the level of pulmonary arterial pressure is determined by systemic arterial pressure, in a small or medium defect the pulmonary arterial pressure is determined by a combination of pulmonary vascular resistance and pulmonary blood flow. In most of these patients the pulmonary vascular resistance falls normally with age. Pulmonary vascular disease can raise the pulmonary vascular resistance in time, but this occurs at a slower rate than with large defects and in only a few patients with a large volume left-to-right shunt. The volume of pulmonary blood flow varies with the size of the defect and the level of pulmonary vascular resistance, and since beyond infancy most children have normal pulmonary vascular resistance, the shunt is directly related to the size of the defect. In some patients the defect is so small that the shunt is undetectable by oximetry data, while in other patients the pulmonary blood flow is three times the systemic blood flow. In most patients, however, the pulmonary blood flow is probably less than twice the volume of systemic blood flow.

History

Most patients with small and medium ventricular septal defects are asymptomatic. Heart disease is usually detected by the discovery of a murmur either prior to discharge from the newborn nursery or, more commonly, at the first postnatal visit to the physician. Those patients with a large pulmonary blood flow may have frequent respiratory infections and pneumonia. A few patients develop congestive cardiac failure. The growth and development of most patients are normal.

Physical Examination

Usually there is no evidence of cardiomegaly on physical examination. A systolic murmur is present along the lower left sternal border and may be associated with a thrill. In very small defects the murmur may appear midsystolic in timing, but in most patients it is pansystolic. In some patients with a small defect, probably that located in the muscular septum, the murmur is grade II/VI in loudness and has a "squirty" quality. Usually, however, the murmurs are grade III-IV/VI in loudness.

As in those patients with large defects, it is important to define pulmonary arterial pressure by the loudness of the pulmonary component of the second sound (P_2) and to define pulmonary blood flow by the presence of an apical diastolic murmur. In patients with a small defect, P_2

is normal and diastole is clear, while those with medium defects may have an accentuated P_2 and a soft apical murmur.

Electrocardiographic Features

In many patients in this category, the electrocardiogram is normal, reflecting that the volume of pulmonary blood flow and level of pulmonary arterial pressure are normal or near normal. A pattern of left ventricular hypertrophy indicates an increased volume of pulmonary blood flow with little change in pulmonary arterial pressure. A few patients with elevation of pulmonary arterial pressure and pulmonary blood flow have a pattern of biventricular hypertrophy.

Roentgenographic Features

The cardiac size, left atrial size, and pulmonary vascularity directly parallel the volume of pulmonary blood flow. The heart and lung fields may be normal or may show increased vascularity and size, but not to the degree found in patients with large ventricular septal defect and blood flow.

Summary of Clinical Findings

In ventricular septal defect, the magnitude of the shunt is dependent upon the size of the defect and the relative levels of pulmonary and systemic vascular resistances. A loud pansystolic murmur along the left sternal border is the hallmark of ventricular septal defect. The other clinical and laboratory findings reflect alterations of hemodynamics. Alterations in the second sound, the presence of an apical diastolic murmur, and changes in the electrocardiogram and roentgenogram variously reflect the magnitude of shunt and the level of pulmonary arterial pressure.

Natural History

Patients with small or medium ventricular septal defect, pulmonary blood flow less than twice systemic blood flow, and normal pulmonary arterial pressure are considered to have a normal life expectancy. They are at risk only for bacterial endocarditis. Some patients with a larger volume of pulmonary blood flow or with elevated pulmonary arterial pressure may develop pulmonary vascular changes.

Cardiac Catheterization

In patients with clinical evidence of an obvious, small ventricular septal defect, cardiac catheterization is not indicated. Cardiac catheterization in the other patients is carried out to verify the diagnois and to determine the volume of pulmonary blood flow and level of pulmonary arterial pressure. Therefore, careful oximetry and pressure data are obtained, but usually angiography is not necessary. In those patients requiring catheterization, the study should ordinarily not be performed before the age of 4 or 5 years, when the child might be considered for operation if the defect is large, and when the likelihood of further decrease in the size of the defect is remote. Catheterization is performed at an earlier age if cardiac failure or other major symptoms develop.

Operative Considerations

The operative mortality and morbidity for patients with a small defect probably exceed the problems that might arise in the unoperated patient. Patients with either elevated pulmonary arterial pressure or pulmonary blood flow twice normal should undergo operative closure. Closure can be performed at a low risk, and eliminates the risk of development of pulmonary vascular disease and bacterial endocarditis.

SUMMARY

In ventricular septal defect, the magnitude of the shunt is dependent upon the size of the defect and the relative levels of pulmonary and systemic vascular resistances. A loud pansystolic murmur along the left sternal border is the hallmark of ventricular septal defect. The other clinical and laboratory findings reflect alterations of hemodynamics. Alterations in the second sound, the presence of an apical diastolic murmur and changes in the electrocardiogram and roentgenogram variously reflect the magnitude of shunt and the level of pulmonary arterial pressure.

Patent Ductus Arteriosus

Patent ductus arteriosus (Fig. 17) represents the persistence of fetal communication between the aorta and the pulmonary trunk. The ductus arteriosus is the embryonic left sixth aortic arch and connects the aorta opposite the left subclavian artery and the proximal left pulmonary artery. Normally the ductus arteriosus functionally closes by 1 day of age. Although the mechanisms for closure of the ductus are largely unknown, oxygen and prostaglandin E are factors influencing its closure.

The direction and magnitude of flow through the ductus depend upon the size of the ductus and the relative systemic and pulmonary vascular resistances. In fetal life the ductus is large, and since the pulmonary vascular resistance exceeds systemic vascular resistance, blood flow is from right to left. Following birth, if the ductus arteriosus remains patent, the shunt occurs from the aorta into the pulmonary artery. In patients with a

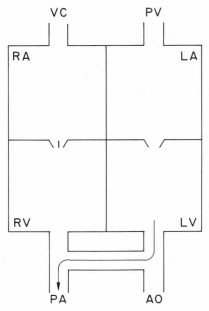

Figure 17. Central circulation in patent ductus arteriosus.

large patent ductus arteriosus, pressures are equal in the aorta and the pulmonary artery, and blood flows into the pulmonary artery because the pulmonary resistance is normally less than systemic resistance. In patients with a smaller ductus arteriosus, the shunt also occurs left to right because of pressure differences between the great vessels.

The hemodynamics resemble ventricular septal defect. As pulmonary vascular resistance falls following birth, the volume of pulmonary blood flow increases. If the volume of pulmonary blood flow is large, congestive cardiac failure occurs because of the excessive volume load placed upon the left ventricle.

History

Patent ductus arteriosus occurs more frequently in females and in prematurely born children. In children whose mothers had rubella during the first trimester of pregnancy, patent ductus arteriosus is the most commonly observed cardiac defect. Patent ductus arteriosus occurs more commonly in children born at high altitudes (above 10,000 ft), emphasizing the role of oxygen in closure of the ductus.

The course of patients with patent ductus arteriosus is variable, depending upon the size of the ductus and the volume of pulmonary blood flow. Many patients are asymptomatic; the ductus is identified only by the presence of a murmur. On the other hand, congestive cardiac failure can develop early in infancy because of volume overload of the left ventricle, although this typically does not occur for at least 3 months. In prematurely born infants, cardiac failure may develop at an earlier age because pulmonary vascular resistance reaches normal levels at an earlier age.

Symptomatic children may also present a history of frequent respiratory infections and easy fatigability.

Physical Examination

The classical physical finding is a continuous or machinery type murmur. Blood flows through the ductus arteriosus throughout the cardiac cycle because of the pressure or resistance difference between the systemic or pulmonary vascular circuits. The murmur may not continue through the entire cardiac cycle, but generally it does extend well into diastole except in the first few months of life. At this age the murmur may be confined to systole, perhaps because the diastolic pressure in the pulmonary artery is similar to that in the aorta.

The murmur is best heard over the upper left chest under the clavicle and may be associated with a thrill or prominent pulsations in the suprasternal notch.

Another set of physical findings related to the blood flow in the pulmonary circulation resembles that of aortic insufficiency. A wide pulse pressure occurs, the systolic pressure being elevated because of an increased stroke volume and the diastolic pressure being lowered because of the flow into the pulmonary circuit. The blood pressure reading shows a wide pulse pressure and peripheral arterial pulses are prominent. In patients with a small patent ductus arteriosus, the blood pressure readings may be normal, but those patients with a larger flow show wide pulse pressure. Radial pulses are usually difficult to palpate in a newborn or small infant. Prominent radial arterial pulses in this age group suggest either ductus arteriosus or coarctation of the aorta. If the femoral pulses are bounding, coarctation is not present.

As in ventricular septal defect, the severity of patent ductus arteriosus may be assessed from two findings: the intensity of the pulmonic component of the second heart sound and the presence of an apical diastolic murmur. The pulmonary component of the second heart sound is accentuated in pulmonary hypertension, whether from increased pulmonary blood flow or from increased pulmonary vascular resistance. An apical diastolic murmur suggests a large left-to-right shunt through the patent ductus arteriosus, resulting in a large volume of blood crossing a normal mitral valve (relative mitral stenosis). Frequently an aortic systolic ejection click is heard because the aorta is dilated.

In an occasional patient the pulmonary resistance exceeds the systemic resistance so that blood flow occurs from the pulmonary artery into the aorta. Such patients have a soft systolic murmur, a loud pulmonic second sound, and differential cyanosis involving the lower extremities.

Electrocardiographic Features

The electrocardiographic patterns in patent ductus arteriosus are similar to those in ventricular septal defect since, in both, the potential hemo-dynamic burdens are volume overload of the left ventricle and pressure overload of the right ventricle. As in patients with ventricular septal defect, one of four patterns may be present. The tracing may be normal in patients with a small patent ductus arteriosus, indicating near normal pulmonary blood flow, pulmonary arterial pressure, and pulmonary vascular resistance. In many patients with patent ductus arteriosus, the major hemodynamic burden is volume overload of the left atrium and left ventricle, the electrocardiogram revealing left ventricular hypertrophy and perhaps left atrial enlargement (Fig. 18). In such patients, pulmonary arterial pressure is near normal. In general, the left ventricular hypertrophy is manifested by a QRS complex in lead V_6 with a sizable Q wave and a very tall R wave followed by a tall T wave. In infants and patients with increased pulmonary arterial pressure, right ventricular hypertrophy co-exists with the pattern of left ventricular hypertrophy. This may be manifested by patterns of left and right ventricular hypertrophy or tall (70 mm)

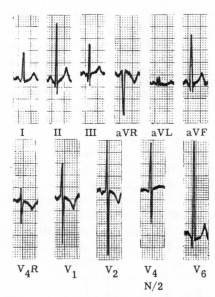

I   II   III   aVR   aVL   aVF

V_4R V_1 V_2 V_4 V_6

N/2

Figure 18. Electrocardiogram in patent ductus arteriosus. Normal QRS axis and P waves. Left ventricular hypertrophy manifested by deep Q wave and tall R wave in lead V_6. N/2 = half-standardization.

equiphasic QRS complexes in the mid-precordial leads. Finally, isolated right ventricular hypertrophy may be present in those patients with a major elevation of pulmonary vascular resistance secondary to pulmonary vascular disease. The elevated resistance reduces pulmonary blood flow so that left ventricular hypertrophy is not present.

Roentgenographic Features

The roentgenographic findings of patent ductus arteriosus typically exhibit increased pulmonary vascularity, and left atrial and left ventricular enlargement. Usually both the aorta and the pulmonary trunk are enlarged, although in infants the aortic knob may be obscured by the thymus. Patent ductus arteriosus is the only major cardiac malformation with a left-to-right shunt with aortic enlargement. The aorta is enlarged because it carries not only the systemic output but also the blood to be shunted through the lungs. In each of the other cardiac malformations discussed in this section on left-to-right shunts, the aorta is normal or appears small. Therefore, if a distinctly enlarged aorta is present and a left-to-right shunt is suspected, patent ductus arteriosus must be seriously considered (Fig. 19).

Cardiac and left atrial size varies from normal to greatly enlarged, depending upon the volume of shunt. A normal-sized heart is found in patients either with a small ductus or with markedly increased pulmonary vascular resistance.

Summary of Clinical Findings

The primary features of patent ductus arteriosus include the continuous murmur and the findings associated with a wide pulse pressure. The

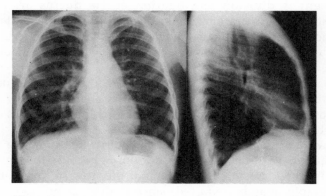

Figure 19. Thoracic roentgenogram of patent ductus arteriosus. Normal-sized heart. Pulmonary vasculature increased. Both aorta and pulmonary artery prominent.

71

secondary features are used to define the relationship $P = R \times F$. Pulmonary arterial pressure is indicated by the intensity of the pulmonic component of the second heart sound and the degree of right ventricular hypertrophy on the electrocardiogram. Flow is reflected by electrocardiographic evidence of left ventricular hypertrophy, the roentgenographic findings of cardiomegaly and left atrial enlargement, or the development of congestive cardiac failure. The presence of an apical diastolic murmur also reflects increased flow but may be obscured by the continuous murmur.

Natural History

The course of patients with patent ductus arteriosus resembles that previously described for patients with ventricular septal defect. Patients with a small or medium patent ductus arteriosus do well and have few complications other than bacterial endocarditis. Pulmonary vascular disease can develop in patients with a large patent ductus arteriosus and those with elevated pulmonary arterial pressure and blood flow. As pulmonary vascular resistance rises, the volume of pulmonary blood flow falls. Eventually the pulmonary vascular resistance can exceed the systemic vascular resistance and the shunt becomes right to left. Such patients have differential cyanosis manifested by cyanosis of the lower extremities and normal color of the upper extremities.

Similarly to patients with ventricular septal defect who develop pulmonary vascular disease, as the pulmonary vascular resistance increases the congestive cardiac failure improves, the diastolic murmur fades, and the left ventricular hypertrophy and cardiomegaly disappear.

Operative Considerations

The treatment is division and ligation of the ductus arteriosus. In asymptomatic cases, operation should be delayed until the child is 1 year old. The ductus should be ligated when the patient is younger if it causes congestive cardiac failure. In older children it should be ligated when recognized.

Considerations concerning the ligation of a ductus in neonates with respiratory distress syndrome are discussed in a later section.

The risk of ligation and division of patent ductus arteriosus is extremely small and the results are generally excellent.

Usually we do not perform cardiac catheterization and angiocardiography in patients with patent ductus arteriosus because the physical and laboratory findings are so characteristic of the disease. In infants, however, aortography may be required, since in this age group the findings may not be as diagnostic, and differentiation from aorticopulmonary window and truncus arteriosus must be made prior to operation in the sick infant.

Summary

Patent ductus arteriosus is an abnormal communication between the aorta and the pulmonary artery. It occurs more frequently in prematurely born females and in infants whose mothers had rubella in the first trimester of pregnancy. The hemodynamics and many clinical findings resemble those of ventricular septal defect because each places an excessive volume of blood on the left ventricle and may elevate pulmonary arterial pressure. The characteristic finding is a continuous murmur and is combined with findings reflecting the flow and pressure characteristics. Ligation and division of the ductus is indicated in almost all patients and is associated with a low risk.

Atrial Septal Defect

Atrial septal defect (Fig. 20) is most frequently located in the area of the fossa ovalis; defects in this location have been termed ostium secundum type defect. Less frequently, atrial septal defect is of the sinus venosus type, being located immediately below the entrance of the superior vena cava into the right atrium. This type may be associated with partial anomalous pulmonary venous connection of the right upper pulmonary veins to the right atrium.

Atrial septal defect should be distinguished from patent foramen ovale, a small opening or potential opening between the atria in the area of the fossa ovalis. In many infants and fewer older patients, the foramen ovale does not anatomically seal and remains a potential communication right to left if the apparatus is competent and the right atrial pressure is elevated. In conditions that raise left atrial pressure or increase left atrial volume, the foramen ovale may be stretched open to the point of incompetence, resulting in a communication that can permit flow of blood from the left atrium to the right atrium because of the higher pressure in the former.

Atrial septal defect is usually large and allows equalization of the atrial pressures. During diastole, pressure is equal in the atria and the ventricles so that the direction and the magnitude of the shunt are dependent upon the relative compliances of the ventricles.

Ventricular compliance is determined by the thickness of the ventricular wall and the stiffness of the myocardium, as might be altered by fibrosis. Normally the right ventricle is more compliant, i.e., more distensible than the left ventricle, since it is much thinner than the left ventricle. When in

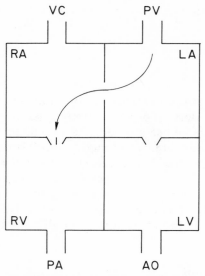

Figure 20. Central circulation in atrial septal defect.

communication at any filling pressure, the right ventricle accepts a greater volume of blood than the left ventricle (Fig. 21).

In most patients with atrial septal defect, the relative ventricular compliances are such to allow a left-to-right shunt through the defect so that the pulmonary blood flow is about three times the systemic blood flow. Factors altering ventricular compliance affect the magnitude and the direction of the shunt. Myocardial fibrosis of the left ventricle, developing from

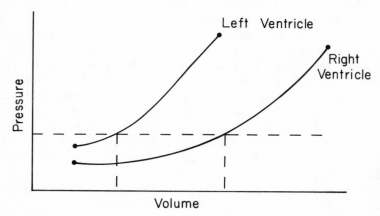

Figure 21. Schematic illustration of relative deficiencies of right and left ventricular compliance.

coronary arterial disease, increases the left-to-right shunt. In contrast, right ventricular hypertrophy, as from pulmonary stenosis, reduces the volume of left-to-right shunt, and if significant, may lead to a right-to-left shunt.

In atrial septal defect the right-sided cardiac chambers and the pulmonary trunk are enlarged. The clinical features of atrial septal defect reflect the enlargement of these chambers and the augmented blood flow through the right-sided cardiac chambers.

In patients with atrial septal defect, the pulmonary arterial pressure is almost always normal during childhood.

History

Several factors obtained in the history may be useful in diagnosing atrial septal defect. Atrial septal defect of the ostium secundum type occurs two to three times more frequently in females.

Children with atrial septal defect rarely develop congestive cardiac failure during infancy and childhood because the major hemodynamic abnormality, volume overload of the right ventricle, is well tolerated. The right ventricle is crescent-shaped and therefore has a large surface area for its resting volume. By altering its shape, the right ventricle can increase its volume without changing myocardial fiber length. According to Laplace's law $T = Pr$, the right ventricle is better able to maintain its pressure volume relationships as the volume increases.

In the right ventricle the pressure (P) is relatively low, while the radius (r) is relatively large. Therefore, although the radius increases the volume, in comparison to the already large radius this increase adds relatively little to the level of tension required to maintain the pressure volume relationship.

On occasion, neonates with atrial septal defect manifest cyanosis in the first week of life and then become acyanotic. The other condition that typically gives such a history is Ebstein's malformation of the tricuspid valve. The transient neonatal cyanosis indicates a right-to-left shunt at the atrial level. Right ventricular compliance in the neonate is decreased because the right ventricle is thick-walled, since prior to birth the right ventricle has developed systemic pressure. The right ventricular hypertrophy alters compliance and leads to a right-to-left shunt (Fig. 21). As pulmonary resistance falls, right ventricular compliance and architecture change, so the shunt becomes left to right.

Typically, the presence of atrial septal defect is first recognized as late as the preschool physical examination because the murmur is soft and may be mistaken for a functional murmur or obscured during the examination of an active or fearful toddler.

Physical Examination

The major cardiac findings are related to increased blood flow through the right side of the heart. Enlargement of the right ventricle may cause a precordial bulge.

The auscultatory features of atrial septal defect are usually diagnostic. The first heart sound in the tricuspid area is accentuated. A systolic murmur is present that results from turbulence due to the increased blood flow across the outflow area of the right ventricle. The murmur is a systolic ejection type and is located in the pulmonary area. The systolic murmur in patients with atrial septal defect varies from grade I-III/VI and is rarely associated with a thrill.

A mid-diastolic murmur caused by increased blood flow across the tricuspid valve is common and is present along the lower left sternal border.

Two characteristics of the second heart sound are important for diagnosis of atrial septal defect. Classically, wide, fixed splitting of the second heart sound is present. Wide splitting results from a marked delay of the pulmonic component because right ventricular ejection is prolonged and related to the increased volume of blood that it must eject. Any condition in which the right ventricle ejects a larger quantity of blood has wide splitting. The second heart sound has also been described as fixed, indicating that no variation occurs in the degree of splitting between inspiration and expiration. Fixed splitting indicates the presence of atrial communication. Because the degree of shunt is determined by the relative ventricular compliances, the relative volume of blood entering each ventricle is constant, regardless of the total volume of blood presented to the atria. During inspiration an increased systemic venous return enters the total volume of blood in the atria, so that during this phase of respiration less blood flows left to right. During expiration, systemic venous return diminishes and the left-to-right shunt increases. But in each state the relative amount of blood entering each ventricle is constant, so duration of ejection for each ventricle is also constant.

Fixed splitting of the second heart sound is diagnostic of an interatrial communication and is present in any cardiac abnormality with an atrial communication. On occasion the murmur may be scarcely audible, but with the fixed splitting of the second heart sound one can make this clinical diagnosis.

The functional pulmonary flow murmur resembles the systolic murmur of atrial septal defect, but it can be distinguished by the presence of a normal second heart sound and the absence of a diastolic murmur.

Electrocardiographic Features

Although the electrocardiogram may be normal in cases of atrial septal defect of the ostium secundum type, it usually reveals abnormalities. The right atrium and right ventricle are anatomically enlarged in atrial septal defect, and the electrocardiogram reflects these changes. Right axis deviation, usually +120° to +150°, is present, and right atrial enlargement is found in many patients.

Right ventricular hypertrophy is also found. The pattern of the QRS complex in lead V_1 is important in the diagnosis of atrial septal defect (Fig. 22). In 95 percent of patients with atrial septal defect, an rsR′ pattern is present in lead V_1, the R′ being tall and broad. Lead V_6 shows a qRs pattern and a prominent and broad S wave. It is difficult to diagnose atrial septal defect in the absence of this electrocardiographic finding.

This particular QRS pattern has also been called incomplete right bundle branch block, but it reflects the increased right ventricular volume. No anatomic abnormality of the conduction system is present. An rSr′ pattern may be found in lead V_1 of some normal children and in some children with other forms of congenital cardiac anomalies not associated with right ventricular enlargement, but the other r′ is neither tall nor broad.

Roentgenographic Features

The chest x-rays, in addition to showing increased pulmonary vascularity, reveal enlargement of the right side of the heart (Fig. 23). On the posteroanterior view, the pulmonary trunk is prominent, as is the right cardiac

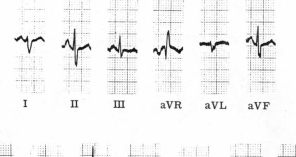

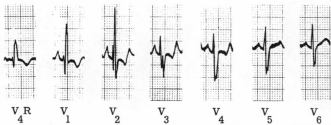

Figure 22. Electrocardiogram in atrial septal defect. QRS axis of 180°. Right atrial enlargement shown by tall peaked P waves in leads V_1 and V_2. rSR′ pattern in leads V_4R and V_1 with broad R′ indicates incomplete right bundle branch block. Right ventricular hypertrophy manifested by large R wave in lead V_1 and deep S wave in lead V_6.

border (right atrium). On the lateral and right anterior oblique views the right ventricle is enlarged. The left atrium is not enlarged since it is readily decompressed by the atrial communication. Therefore, the absence of displacement of the esophagus in the presence of increased pulmonary blood flow indicates an atrial communication.

Summary of Clinical Findings

In atrial septal defect, the fixed splitting of the second heart sound indicates the presence of an atrial communication. The other findings— pulmonary ejection murmur, tricuspid diastolic murmur, rsR' on electrocardiogram, cardiomegaly and increased pulmonary blood flow—each reflect the augmented volume of flow through the right side of the heart. In virtually all patients with atrial septal defect, the flow through the right side of the heart is about three times normal and the pulmonary arterial pressure is normal. Thus, assessment of the severity of the condition is of less concern than in the case of most other forms of left-to-right shunts.

Natural History

Children with atrial septal defect rarely develop pulmonary arterial hypertension and are usually asymptomatic. In adulthood the incidence of pulmonary vascular disease increases with each decade, although it rarely reaches the degree found in patients with ventricular septal defect or patent ductus arteriosus. Ultimately, tricuspid insufficiency develops and leads to cardiac failure, atrial arrhythmias, and development of right-to-left shunt. The average life span of those with untreated atrial septal defect is in the mid-fifties.

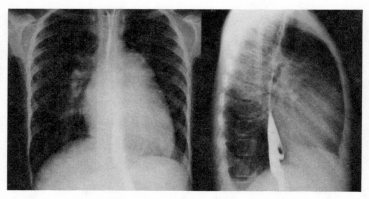

Figure 23. Thoracic roentgenogram in atrial septal defect. Left. Posteroanterior view. Cardiomegaly and increased pulmonary blood flow; enlarged pulmonary artery segment. Right. Lateral view. Enlargement of right ventricle indicated by obliteration of retrosternal space. No displacement of barium-filled esophagus.

One interesting fact of atrial septal defect is the rarity of bacterial endocarditis, probably because of the absence of jet lesions in this condition and the fact that there is no significant pressure gradient between the atria. Therefore, patients with atrial septal defect of the secundum type are the one group of patients with congenital cardiac disease who do not require prophylaxis for endocarditis.

Cardiac Catheterization

Cardiac catheterization reveals a large increase in oxygen saturation at the atrial level from the left-to-right shunt; this is maintained throughout the right side of the heart. In children the pulmonary arterial pressure is almost always normal. A pressure gradient of 10 to 20 mm Hg may be present between the right ventricle and the pulmonary artery, caused by increased blood flow and not by an anatomic obstructive condition. The atrial pressures are equal and the left atrial pressure is lower than normal.

Often cardiac catheterization is combined with pulmonary arteriography. If contrast material is injected into the pulmonary artery, the pulmonary veins fill after 2 or 3 seconds. A coexistent anomalous pulmonary venous connection may be identified by this means, although the distinction of the precise site of drainage may be difficult.

Operative Considerations

In most children with clinically recognizable atrial septal defect, the defect should be operatively closed. Although the operation requires cardiopulmonary bypass, the operative risk is very low. Usually the hospital stay is brief. There are few patients with long-term complications, usually an arrhythmia. Patients with an atrial septal defect and pulmonary blood flow less than twice normal do not require operation. The optimum age for operation is between 5 and 10 years of age.

Summary

Atrial septal defect occurs more frequently in females, is recognized later in life than most forms of congenital cardiac disease, and rarely results in cardiac failure in the pediatric age range. Physical examination, laboratory findings, and roentgenograms are usually sufficient to diagnose the condition. Large atrial septal defects should be operatively closed during childhood, to prevent complications in adulthood.

Endocardial Cushion Defect

Endocardial cushion defect (Fig. 24) is a general term for a group of cardiac malformations that include a range of defects in the formation of the endocardial cushions. Developmentally, the endocardial cushions contribute to the lower portion of the atrial septum, the upper portion of the ventricular septum, and the septal leaflets of the mitral and tricuspid valves. Therefore, defective development of various portions of the endocardial cushions can result in several types of malformations. The defects classified in this group actually represent a spectrum of malformations. The simplest malformation, *ostium primum defect* or incomplete atrioventricular canal, consists of an atrial septal defect located low in the atrial septum, adjacent to the mitral valve annulus, which is often associated with a cleft in the anterior leaflet of the mitral valve, leading to mitral insufficiency. In other cases the ostium primum type defect is continuous with a larger defect in the ventricular septum. In these instances the defect crosses both the mitral valvular annulus and the tricuspid valvular annulus, leading to deficiencies of the septal leaflets of both the tricuspid and mitral valves. This form of endocardial cushion defect is called *complete atrioventricular canal*.

There are three major hemodynamic abnormalities. The first is the volume overload on the right atrium and right ventricle, as in patients with a left-to-right shunt at the atrial level. Even if the endocardial cushion defect involves portions of the ventricular septum, more of the shunt occurs above the level of the atrioventricular valves, and thus at the atrial level. The second abnormality is mitral insufficiency that leads to increased left ventricular volume because the left ventricle handles not only the normal cardiac output but also the regurgitated volume. In contrast to the usual patient with a mitral insufficiency, left atrial enlargement is usually not

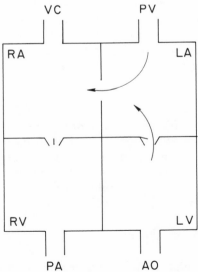

Figure 24. Central circulation in endocardial cushion defect.

present, because the left atrium is really decompressed by the atrial septal communication. The third abnormality relates to the varying degrees of pulmonary hypertension. Generally, the more deficient the ventricular septum, the higher the level of pulmonary arterial pressure, even though there may be little ventricular shunt. The pulmonary hypertension is related to varying contributions of pulmonary vascular resistance and blood flow.

History

The histories of patients with endocardial cushion defect vary considerably. In general, symptoms appear earlier in patients with more extensive endocardial cushion defect and abnormalities of the mitral valve. Infants with the complete form of atrioventricular canal frequently develop congestive cardiac failure in the first few weeks or months of life, whereas patients with the ostium primum type defect may be asymptomatic as a ostium secundum type atrial septal defect.

When present, the symptoms are usually those related to congestive cardiac failure, poor growth, and frequent respiratory infections. Mild cyanosis may be related to right-to-left shunt either from the streaming of inferior vena caval blood through the defect or from the development of pulmonary vascular disease. Frequently, the murmur is heard early in life, even if the patient is asymptomatic. Down's syndrome (trisomy 21) is frequently found in association with endocardial cushion defect. Therefore, in dealing with a child with this particular trisomic condition and cardiac disease, the first diagnostic consideration is endocardial cushion defect.

Physical Examination

The general appearance of the child may be normal, but infants with congestive cardiac failure may be scrawny, dyspneic and tachypneic. In patients with cardiac enlargement, the precordial bulges and the cardiac apex are displaced toward the left and inferiorly.

The auscultatory findings vary, but characteristically they reflect mitral insufficiency and left-to-right shunt at the atrial level. In patients with ostium primum defect and cleft mitral valve, five findings may be present. 1. Apical pansystolic murmur of mitral insufficiency. This murmur radiates to the axilla and may be associated with a thrill. The absence of a murmur of mitral insufficiency does not preclude a cleft mitral valve. 2. Apical mid-diastolic murmur. This murmur is present in patients with larger amounts of mitral insufficiency. 3. Pulmonary systolic ejection murmur. This murmur is similar in characteristics and origin to the pulmonary flow murmur of atrial septal defect of the ostium secundum type.

4. Wide, fixed splitting of S_2. The second cardiac sound reveals these characteristic findings. The pulmonic component of the second sound may be accentuated if associated pulmonary hypertension coexists. 5. Tricuspid diastolic murmur. Because of the left-to-right shunt at the atrial level, a large blood flow crosses the tricuspid valve.

Although these are the expected findings, in some patients a murmur of ventricular septal defect is found. A few patients with pulmonary vascular disease, surprisingly, have minor murmurs, but the pulmonic component of the second heart sound is accentuated.

Electrocardiographic Features

The electrocardiogram in endocardial cushion defect is diagnostic (Fig. 25). Five features are commonly observed: 1) left axis deviation, 2) prolonged PR interval, 3) atrial enlargement, 4) ventricular hypertrophy, and 5) rSR' pattern in lead V_1. The first two features are related to the abnormal position of the conduction system in the ventricle. The bundle of His is displaced inferiorly by the defect and enters along the posterior aspect of the ventricular septum. Ventricular depolarization proceeds inferiorly to superiorly and generally leftward. This leads to left axis deviation. The QRS axis may range from 0° to −150°; greater degrees of left axis deviation occur in patients with increasing degrees of right ventricular hypertrophy, secondary to elevated pulmonary arterial pressure. The prolonged PR interval is probably related to the longer course of the bundle of His.

The last three features reflect the cardiac hemodynamics and vary according to the relative volume and the pressure loads on the respective ventricles. They are therefore helpful in assessing the hemodynamic characteristics of the particular defect. Right atrial enlargement is usually present. Often biventricular hypertrophy is present, left ventricular hypertrophy indicating excess volume in the left ventricle and right ventricular hypertrophy arising from combinations of excess right ventricular volume and increased pulmonary arterial pressure. Often an rSR' pattern is found in lead V_1 because of increased right ventricular volume. Despite the abnormal ventricular conduction sequence, the precordial leads accurately predict ventricular hypertrophy.

Roentgenographic Features

In addition to the increase in pulmonary vascularity, varying degrees of cardiomegaly are observed. Cardiac size is increased because of the left-to-right shunt and also the mitral insufficiency with its resultant left ventricular enlargement. As a result of the mitral insufficiency, the heart is often enlarged out of proportion, due to increased pulmonary vascular markings (Fig. 26). Left atrial enlargement may be present, although it is

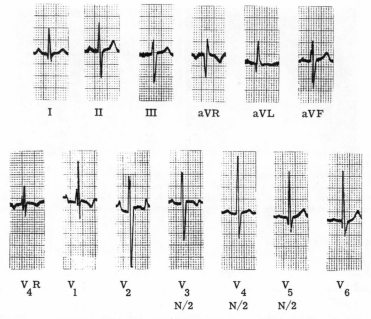

Figure 25. Electrocardiogram of endocardial cushion defect. QRS axis of $-30°$. Biventricular hypertrophy. rSR' pattern in lead V_1. N/2 = half-standardization.

not as prominent as that observed in ventricular septal defect with a shunt of comparable magnitude. The right-sided cardiac chambers are also enlarged.

Summary of Clinical Findings

Although the clinical and laboratory findings vary considerably, the electrocardiographic features are the most diagnostic for endocardial cushion defect. The auscultatory, electrocardiographic, and roentgenographic findings reflect the three potential hemodynamic abnormalities: mitral insufficiency, pulmonary hypertension, and left-to-right shunt at the atrial level.

Natural History

Patients with complete endocardial cushion defect develop intractable cardiac failure in infancy and present a difficult management problem. They also develop pulmonary vascular disease during childhood. Patients with an ostium primum defect and mild mitral insufficiency are asymptomatic into adulthood.

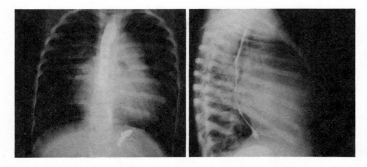

Figure 26. Thoracic roentgenogram of endocardial cushion defect. Left. Posteroanterior view. Cardiomegaly and increased pulmonary vasculature. Prominent right atrium and pulmonary arterial segment. Right. Lateral view. Slight displacement of barium-filled esophagus. Retrosternal space filled in by prominent right ventricle and pulmonary artery.

Cardiac Catheterization

At cardiac catheterization a large increase in oxygen saturation is found at the atrial level. Occasionally an additional increase is found at the ventricular level, but the atrial increase is so large it obscures the ventricular component of the shunt. The pulmonary arterial pressure ranges from normal to systemic levels, the latter suggesting a complete atrioventricular canal. There may also be a slight right-to-left atrial shunt.

Left ventriculography reveals a characteristic abnormality of the left ventricle termed goose-neck deformity. The medial border of the left ventricle, when viewed on an anteroposterior film, appears scooped out because of the lower margin of the endocardial cushion defect and the presence of abnormal chordal attachment to the septum. Mitral insufficiency is also demonstrated by the study and a left-to-right shunt.

Operative Considerations

In patients who are asymptomatic or have few symptoms, the operation can be delayed until the age of 5 to 10 years. Most of such patients have an ostium primum type defect and a cleft mitral valve, and operation can be performed at a low risk. The defect is closed and frequently the cleft of the mitral valve is sutured. Plastic repair of the mitral valve may greatly reduce the degree of mitral insufficiency.

In patients with complete atrioventricular canal, corrective operation can be carried out, at a higher risk; frequently the patients require replacement of the mitral valve. Decisions are difficult to make in symptomatic infants, who often respond poorly to medical management. Banding of the pulmonary artery is beneficial in a few instances. The other option, corrective operation, carries a high risk because of the infant's size and the difficulties encountered in repair or replacement of the mitral valve.

Summary

Endocardial cushion defect encompasses a group of anomalies involving specific portions of the atrial and ventricular septae and adjacent atrioventricular valves. The clinical and laboratory findings reflect the atrial left-to-right shunt and the mitral regurgitation in this patient. The electrocardiogram showing left axis deviation, atrial and ventricular hypertrophy, and incomplete right bundle branch block is quite diagnostic. X-ray studies reveal enlargement of each cardiac chamber. The anatomic features of the defect complicate operative correction.

Summary of Left-to-Right Shunts

Certain generalizations can be made concerning the cardiac conditions with left-to-right shunts that aid in understanding their hemodynamics and can be applied to other lesions, such as those with admixture.

Shunts occurring distal to the mitral valve have certain general characteristics. The flow through the defect is dependent upon either the size of the defect or the relative resistances of the pulmonary and systemic vascular systems. Therefore, the systolic events influence the shunt primarily. Volume load is placed upon the left side of the heart and can lead to congestive cardiac failure. Left atrial enlargement, apical diastolic murmur, and left ventricular hypertrophy are other manifestations of the excess volume in the left side of the heart.

Shunts occurring proximal to the mitral valve have other characteristics. The shunt is dependent upon the relative compliance of the ventricles and therefore is influenced predominantly by the diastolic events. Congestive heart failure is uncommon in uncomplicated cardiac defects because the volume load is placed on the right ventricle. Left atrial enlargement is absent. The electrocardiogram shows a pattern of right ventricular volume overload, and a tricuspid diastolic murmur may be present.

The features and classic findings of the four major acyanotic conditions associated with increased pulmonary blood flow are presented in Table 8.

OBSTRUCTIVE LESIONS

While conditions leading to obstruction to blood flow from the heart are common in children, those causing inflow obstruction, such as mitral stenosis, are comparatively rare. In this section, therefore, the emphasis will be upon aortic stenosis, pulmonary stenosis, and coarctation of the aorta.

TABLE 8. SUMMARY OF DEFECTS WITH ACYANOSIS AND INCREASED PULMONARY BLOOD FLOW (LEFT-TO-RIGHT SHUNT)

	HISTORY				PHYSICAL EXAMINATION			
Malformation	Sex Incidence	Major Associated Syndrome	Congestive Cardiac Failure	Age Murmur First Heard	Pulse Pressure	Thrill	Murmur	Degree Splitting of S_2
Atrial septal defect	F > M	None	Rare	5 yrs	Normal	Rare	Grade I-III ejection systolic murmur pulmonary area Tricuspid diastolic rumble	Fixed, wide splitting
Ventricular septal defect	F = M	None	± 3-8 mo	6 wks	Normal	Precordial	Grade IV harsh pansystolic left sternal border Diastolic rumble	Normal
Patent ductus arteriosus	F > M	Rubella Low birth rate	± 3-8 mo	Infancy	Wide	Upper precordial (±) Suprasternal notch (±)	Machinery type or systolic (infant) Apical diastolic rumble	Normal
Endocardial cushion defect	F = M	Down's	±	Infancy	Normal	Apical (±)	Grade I-IV apical pansystolic murmur ejection systolic murmur pulmonary area Tricuspid rumble	Fixed, wide splitting

Malformation	ELECTROCARDIOGRAM				ROENTGENOGRAM	
	Axis	Atrial Enlargement	Ventricular Hypertrophy	Other	Left Atrial Enlargement	Aortic Enlargement
Atrial septal defect	Normal or right	None or right	Right	Incomplete RBBB (rSR´-V$_1$)	Absent	Absent
Ventricular septal defect	Normal or right	None or left	Left (small defect) Biventricular (medium defect) Right (high pulmonary vascular resistance)	None	Present	Absent
Patent ductus arteriosus	Normal	None or left	As above	None	Present	Present
Endocardial cushion defect	Left	Right, left or both	Biventricular	Incomplete RBBB (rSR´-V$_1$) First degree heart block	Present	Absent

F = female
M = male
mo = months
RBBB = right bundle branch block
S$_2$ = second heart sound

wks = weeks
yrs = years
± = may be present or absent
> = greater than

87

Each of these conditions has the following two major effects upon the circulation. 1. Blood flow through the obstruction is turbulent. The turbulence leads to both a systolic ejection type murmur and dilatation of the great vessel beyond the obstruction. 2. The systolic pressure is elevated proximal to the obstruction, and this leads to myocardial hypertrophy, the degree of hypertrophy being proportional to the degree of obstruction. The severity of obstruction varies considerably among patients, but the smaller the orifice size, the greater the level of pressure required to deliver the cardiac output past the obstruction:

$$\text{Orifice size} = K \; \frac{\text{Cardiac output}}{\text{Pressure difference across obstruction}}$$

The primary response to the obstruction is myocardial hypertrophy and not ventricular dilatation. During childhood the heart usually maintains the elevated ventricular pressure without dilatation; however, eventually ventricular enlargement may develop because of the development of myocardial fibrosis. Such fibrotic changes in the ventricle occur because of an imbalance between the myocardial oxygen demands and supply. In most children, coronary arterial blood flow is normal, but with ventricular hypertrophy, myocardial oxygen requirements are increased.

Myocardial oxygen requirements are largely devoted to the development of myocardial tension, and therefore are related directly to the level of ventricular systolic pressure and the number of times per minute the heart must develop that level of pressure. Thus, elevated ventricular systolic pressure and tachycardia increase myocardial oxygen consumption. When a patient with an obstructive lesion exercises, severe increases in myocardial oxygen requirements occur for two reasons. 1. During exercise, cardiac output increases; ergo, according to the relationship shown on the previous page, ventricular systolic pressure also increases. 2. With exercise, the heart rate increases. If these increased myocardial oxygen requirements cannot be met, myocardial ischemia occurs, and ultimately can lead to myocardial fibrosis. These myocardial changes occur over a period of time and can lead to signs and symptoms. With the development of sufficient fibrosis, the contractile properties of the ventricle are affected so that ventricular dilatation and cardiac enlargement develop.

As a group, the obstructive conditions are associated with normal pulmonary vascularity because the cardiac output is normal.

Children with obstructive lesions usually show few symptoms, but severe degrees of obstruction lead to congestive cardiac failure in infancy.

Coarctation of the Aorta

Coarctation of the aorta (Fig. 27) is a narrowing of the descending aorta that usually occurs in the region of the ductus arteriosus. Coarctation has been classified in several ways, but it is best defined by its relationship to the ductus arteriosus (either patent or ligamentous). It can be described as either preductal or postductal. Furthermore, coarctation may occur as either a localized constriction of the aorta or as tubular hypoplasia of the distal aortic arch and proximal descending aorta. The latter form may also coexist with localized coarctation. In general, patients with tubular hypoplasia of the aortic arch develop cardiac failure in infancy. This type of coarctation may be associated with a patent ductus arteriosus located beyond the aortic narrowing and a right-to-left shunt through the ductus arteriosus. The coarctation in older children is usually localized and is postductal in location. The aorta beyond the coarctation shows poststenotic dilatation. In at least 50 percent of patients, a bicuspid aortic valve coexists.

Coarctation of the aorta offers mechanical obstruction to blood flow from the heart. The pressure proximal to the coarctation is elevated, while that beyond the obstruction is lower than normal; this blood pressure difference is the major diagnostic feature of this condition. In response to the pressure difference between the proximal and distal compartments of the aorta, collateral arterial vessels develop between the high pressure ascending portions and the low pressure descending portions of the aorta.

Collateral vessels develop in any vascular system when a pressure difference exists. These are naturally occurring small arteries bridging the high and low pressure components. Blood flows through these bridging

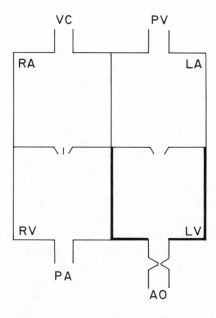

Figure 27. Central circulation in coarctation of aorta.

vessels, the volume of flow slowly increasing, and eventually the vessels dilate. The internal mammary and intercostal arteries are the most frequently occurring collateral vessels in coarctation of the aorta.

Left ventricular hypertrophy develops in response to the elevated systolic pressure proximal to the coarctation.

History

Although most children with coarctation of the aorta are asymptomatic throughout childhood, 10 percent develop congestive cardiac failure during infancy. In the latter group, recognition of the lesion is important because proper management can be lifesaving. Older children rarely develop congestive cardiac failure, but rather have complaints, such as headaches, related to the systemic hypertension in the upper portion of the body. The ominous sign of chest pain may be present occasionally, and indicates myocardial ischemia secondary to left ventricular hypertrophy.

In coarctation of the aorta, there is a male predominance of 5 to 1. When a diagnosis of coarctation of the aorta is made in a female, one must strongly consider the presence of Turner's syndrome and should perform chromosomal analysis when appropriate.

If coarctation of the aorta does not lead to congestive cardiac failure, the condition is often not recognized until preschool age when the murmur is heard, or at a later age when hypertension is detected.

Physical Examination

Most patients show normal growth and development; many have an athletic physique. In neonates or infants, the signs of congestive cardiac failure may be present and profound. Mild degrees of cyanosis and mottling of the skin may be present because of pulmonary edema and poor perfusion.

Clinical diagnosis of coarctation of the aorta rests on the recognition of a blood pressure differential between the upper and lower extremities. This information may be gathered by palpation of both the radial and the femoral arteries. If there is a substantial difference between the two, one could suspect coarctation of the aorta. In addition, finding very sharp and brisk radial pulses in infants should lead one to consider the diagnosis of coarctation of the aorta; the radial pulses are ordinarily difficult to palpate in this age group. Regardless of whether the femoral pulses feel diminished or not, the blood pressure should be taken in both arms and a leg in any child with a cardiac murmur. Many cases of coarctation of the aorta have been missed because "the femoral arteries were palpable." The blood pressure may be obtained by the flush method, by direct auscultatory means, or with the aid of a Doppler. Blood pressure cuffs of appropriate width must be used. The largest cuff that fits the extremity should be used. In a patient without cardiac disease, the blood pressure should be the same in the upper and lower extremities. If the blood pressure is higher, by 20 mm Hg or more, in the arms than in the legs, this difference is considered significant and diagnostic of coarctation of the aorta.

In infants with congestive cardiac failure secondary to severe coarctation of the aorta, the blood pressure values may be similar in the arms and legs, but at extremely low levels at both sites, because the cardiac output is so reduced. Following digitalization of such infants, however, the pressure difference between the upper and lower extremities usually becomes apparent.

The examination of the heart may reveal cardiac enlargement. Palpation in the suprasternal notch reveals a prominent aortic pulsation and, perhaps, a thrill in patients with coexistent bicuspid aortic valve. An ejection type murmur is present along the sternal border, at the apex, and over the back between the scapulae. The murmur is generally of grade II-III/VI intensity. An aortic systolic ejection click is often heard, indicating dilation of the ascending aorta from the coexistent bicuspid aortic valve. The aortic component of the second heart sound may be increased in intensity. In the infant with congestive cardiac failure, auscultatory findings may be muffled until after digitalization.

Electrocardiographic Features

The electrocardiographic findings vary with the age of the patient. In the neonatal and early infant periods, the electrocardiogram usually reveals right ventricular hypertrophy. There are several explanations for this seemingly paradoxical finding. If the coarctation of the aorta is located beyond the insertion of the patent ductus arteriosus, the right ventricle, because of its communication through the pulmonary artery and ductus arteriosus, is working against the resistance imposed by the coarctation of the aorta. In other patients with coarctation of the aorta and patent ductus arteriosus, the left ventricle is hypoplastic, so the electrocardiogram shows a pattern of right ventricular hypertrophy. Right ventricular hypertrophy has also been explained on the basis of pulmonary hypertension developing secondary to left ventricular failure.

Regardless of its origin, the typical pattern of coarctation of the aorta in a symptomatic infant is right ventricular hypertrophy and inverted T waves in the left precordial leads. Subsequently, the electrocardiogram in these infants shifts to a pattern of left ventricular hypertrophy. In older infants with severe coarctation of the aorta or in those with coexistent endocardial fibroelastosis of the left ventricle, a pattern of left ventricular hypertrophy and inverted T waves and ST depression in the left precordial leads is present. These abnormalities of ventricular repolarization are often signs of a poor prognosis.

In the older patient with coarctation of the aorta, the precordial leads show either left ventricular hypertrophy or a normal pattern.

Roentgenographic Features

In symptomatic infants, significant cardiac enlargement is present, the cardiomegaly consisting primarily of left ventricular and left atrial enlargement. The lung fields show a diffuse reticular pattern of pulmonary edema and pulmonary venous congestion.

In older children the heart size and pulmonary vasculature are normal. The roentgenographic appearance of the descending aorta is often diagnostic of coarctation of the aorta by showing poststenotic dilatation. The barium swallow shows an E sign. The upper portion of the E is formed by the segment of the aorta proximal to the coarctation, and the lower portion of the E is formed by the deviation of the barium by the poststenotic dilatation. Often the left side of the aorta shows soft tissue densities in the form of the number 3, the upper portion of the 3 representing the aortic knob, and the lower portion representing the poststenotic dilatation. These roentgenographic findings help identify the extent of the coarctation. The ascending aorta may be prominent if a bicuspid aortic valve coexists.

In children more than 10 years of age, rib notching may be apparent. The inferior margins of the upper ribs show scalloping, caused by pressure from enlarged intercostal arteries that are serving as collaterals.

Summary of Clinical Findings

Whether the patient is an infant in congestive cardiac failure or an asymptomatic patient, the clinical diagnosis rests upon the demonstration of a blood pressure difference between the arms and leg. Other findings such as those on electrocardiography and thoracic roentgenograms reflect the severity of the condition. Prominence of the ascending aorta on thoracic roentgenogram and apical systolic ejection click indicate a coexistent bicuspid aortic valve.

Cardiac Catheterization and Angiography

Usually the clinical findings are sufficient to diagnose coarctation of the aorta, so catheterization and angiography are not necessary. To obtain information to make operative decisions, one must know the exact location of the coarctation of the aorta. The distal extent of the coarctation can be recognized by the roentgenographic identification of poststenotic dilatation, and the proximal extent by the blood pressure in the two arms. Usually the recordings are similar in both arms, indicating that the coarctation is located distal to the left subclavian artery. Occasionally, the blood pressure of the left arm is lower than in the right arm, indicating that the coarctation of the aorta involves the organ of the left subclavian artery and, therefore, a longer segment of the aorta.

In an infant in cardiac failure, the diagnosis may be difficult, in which case aortography is indicated. Similarly, in the older child without well visualized poststenotic dilatation on thoracic roentgenograms, aortography is required to outline the extent of the coarctation.

Operative Considerations

Operation should be performed on most patients with coarctation of the aorta, although age at operation varies according to the clinical status of the patient. Usually operation should be deferred until the patient is 8 to 10 years of age, provided he is asymptomatic and not hypertensive. If the patient is hypertensive (arm pressure greater than 150/90 mm Hg), operation should be performed by the age of 4 to 5 years or sooner. The operative risk is low (1 percent) in these patients.

Infants with coarctation of the aorta who develop congestive cardiac failure and respond fully to medical management should be carefully followed and operated on at a later time. Infants who fail to respond fully and promptly to medical management require operative repair, often as an emergency procedure. The operative risk is higher in this group.

Natural History

The anastomotic site following coarctation repair may not grow proportionately to the growth of the aortic diameter. Therefore, *recoarctation* may develop, often necessitating a second operation when the patient is older. This need occurs more frequently among children operated on in infancy, but is a small price for a lifesaving procedure. Follow-up of these operated patients should include periodic determination of blood pressure in both the upper and lower extremities. Since half of the patients with coarctation of the aorta have a bicuspid aortic valve, they are at risk for development of bacterial endocarditis. The long-term course of patients with bicuspid aortic valve is unknown because the valve may become insufficient or stenotic with age, and at a future time they may require valvular surgery.

Following operation, some patients have persistent hypertension in both the arms and the legs. The reason for this is unknown and the long-term history is yet to be defined. The hypertension may require treatment.

Summary

Coarctation of the aorta is usually an easily diagnosed condition. In most patients it requires treatment, for it can lead to several problems: congestive cardiac failure, hypertension, and left ventricular fibrosis. In most patients, operation is required to relieve the obstruction. Despite the apparent anatomic success of the operation, recoarctation, persistent hypertension, and coexistent bicuspid aortic valve are long-term problems following it.

Aortic Stenosis

Aortic stenosis can occur at one of three anatomic locations. Most frequently aortic stenosis is caused by a stenotic congenital unicuspid or bicuspid valve. Obstruction to left ventricular outflow may also occur below the aortic valve, either as an isolated fibrous ring (discrete membranous subaortic stenosis) or as septal hypertrophy (idiopathic hypertrophic subaortic stenosis). Aortic stenosis is rarely located in the proximal ascending aorta; it is then called supravalvular aortic stenosis.

Regardless of the site of obstruction, the effect upon the left ventricle is similar. Because of the stenosis, the left ventricular pressure rises to maintain a normal cardiac output. This relationship can be illustrated by the formula used to calculate the severity of valvular aortic stenosis:

$$AVA = \frac{SEP \times HR}{K \sqrt{LVSP-AO}}$$

AVA = aortic valve area (area of stenotic orifice)
LVSP = mean left ventricular ejection pressure
  AO = mean aortic ejection pressure
   K = constant
 SEP = systolic ejection period
  HR = heart rate

In patients with more severe aortic stenosis (smaller aortic valve area) for a given cardiac output (CO), left ventricular systolic pressure is higher. Similarly, when the patient exercises, since the aortic valve area remains unchanged, the cardiac output rises and so does the left ventricular systolic pressure.

The primary effect upon the heart of each type of aortic stenosis is elevation of left ventricular systolic pressure, resulting in left ventricular hypertrophy. Many of the clinical and laboratory features of aortic stenosis are related to the left ventricular hypertrophy and its effects. Because of the elevated left ventricular systolic pressure, the myocardial oxygen demands are increased. During exercise the oxygen demands are further increased because both heart rate and left ventricular systolic pressure increase. If these oxygen needs are unmet, myocardial ischemia may occur and lead to syncope, chest pain, or electrocardiogram changes. Recurrent myocardial ischemic episodes can lead to left ventricular fibrosis, which can ultimately progress to cardiac failure and cardiomegaly.

Another set of clinical features of aortic stenosis are related to the turbulence of blood flow through the stenotic area. Manifested by a systolic ejection murmur, this turbulence can also lead to poststenotic dilatation in valvular aortic stenosis.

AORTIC VALVULAR STENOSIS

Aortic valvular stenosis (Fig. 28) is related to a unicuspid valve in infants and to a congenitally bicuspid valve in older children and adults. The orifices of these abnormal valves are narrowed. In some patients these valves may permit mild degrees of aortic insufficiency.

History

Aortic stenosis is commonly associated with a significant murmur at birth. In most other congenital cardiac conditions, the murmur is first recognized later in infancy or childhood. Aortic stenosis occurs more frequently in males.

Patients with aortic stenosis are usually asymptomatic throughout childhood, even when stenosis is severe. In 5 percent of children with aortic stenosis, congestive cardiac failure develops in the first year of life,

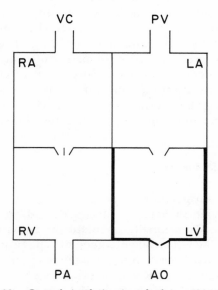

Figure 28. Central circulation in valvular aortic stenosis.

but it uncommonly develops later in childhood. Some of the asymptomatic children, as they approach adolescence, may develop episodes of chest pain having the characteristics of angina. These episodes signify myocardial ischemia and may precede sudden death.

Syncope is another serious symptom of patients with aortic stenosis and may occur upon exercise. The reason for this symptom is largely unknown, but it can be associated with sudden death.

Physical Examination

Several clinical findings suggest the diagnosis of aortic valvular stenosis. In severe stenotic lesions the pulse pressure is narrow and the peripheral pulse feels weak, but in most patients the pulses are normal. A thrill may be present in the aortic area along the upper sternal border and in the suprasternal notch.

An aortic ejection murmur is present, beginning after the first heart sound and extending to the aortic component of the second sound. In older children the murmur is located in the aortic area, but in infancy it is most prominent along the left sternal border; because of its location it may be confused with the murmur of ventricular septal defect. The murmur of aortic stenosis characteristically transmits into the neck vessels. Remember, however, that in nearly every normal child a systolic arterial bruit may be heard over the arterial vessels of the neck, so that the murmur in the neck does not itself prove the diagnosis of aortic valvular stenosis.

The murmur usually follows a systolic ejection click that reflects post-stenotic dilatation of the aorta. Aortic ejection clicks are heard best at the apex of the heart when the patient is reclining. The click is generally present in milder degrees of aortic stenosis, but it may be absent in patients with severe stenosis. In about 30 percent of children with aortic stenosis, a soft, early diastolic murmur of aortic insufficiency may be heard along the upper left sternal border. This is due to minimal reflux of blood from the aorta into the left ventricle secondary to features of the aortic valve.

Electrocardiographic Features

The electrocardiogram generally reveals a normal axis, but in a few patients left axis deviation may be observed, indicating left ventricular myocardial fibrosis. Occasionally in infants and less frequently in older children, there may be left atrial enlargement. The prominent findings are those of left ventricular hypertrophy, usually manifested by deep S waves in lead V_1 and normal or tall R waves in lead V_6.

The electrocardiogram is the most crucial laboratory examination in following the course of children with aortic stenosis. Attention should be directed to serial changes in the ST segment and T waves in precordial leads V_5 and V_6 (Fig. 29). The development of T wave inversion and ST segment depression indicates increasing left ventricular hypertrophy and strain. The presence of left ventricular strain is a warning to the physician; the few children with aortic stenosis who die suddenly usually manifest these electrocardiographic changes of abnormal ventricular repolarization.

Roentgenographic Features

The cardiac size is normal in most children with aortic stenosis because the volume of blood in the heart is normal. Cardiomegaly occurs in infants with severe stenosis and congestive cardiac failure, but it rarely occurs in older children; when present, it indicates fibrotic changes in the left ventricular myocardium. Severe stenosis may be present with a normal cardiac size.

The ascending aorta is prominent, due to poststenotic dilatation. The pulmonary vasculature is normal.

Summary of Clinical Findings

The aortic ejection murmur indicates that the site of the obstruction is in the left ventricular outflow area. The presence of a systolic ejection click and prominent ascending aorta on thoracic roentgenogram reflect poststenotic dilatation of the ascending aorta. The electrocardiogram shows the left ventricular hypertrophy. Chest pain, syncope, ST and T wave changes, and cardiomegaly are serious findings, indicating inadequate myocardial oxygen supply.

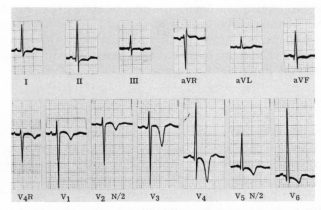

Figure 29. Electrocardiogram in valvular aortic stenosis. Normal QRS axis and P waves. Left ventricular hypertrophy indicated by deep S wave in lead V_1 and tall R wave in lead V_6. Inverted T waves in left precordial leads. N/2 = half-standardization.

97

Natural History

Aortic valvular stenosis may be a progressive condition. Two processes probably account for the progression: the development of myocardial fibrosis, and the decrease in size of the stenotic aortic valvular orifice by cartilaginous changes and ultimately calcification of the valve.

Patients with mild aortic stenosis may live 50 years before they develop symptoms. Such cases represent the calcific aortic stenosis syndrome of adulthood.

Cardiac Catheterization

The oxygen data are usually normal. The important finding is a systolic pressure difference across the aortic valve (Fig. 30). This gradient reflects the degree of obstruction, but to adequately assess the severity, cardiac output must also be considered, as the gradient depends upon the cardiac output. During cardiac catheterization, the measurements of both the pressures and cardiac output should be made simultaneously; with this data the size of the stenotic orifice can be calculated according to the formula on page 94. Aortography or left ventriculography is routinely performed to show the details of the aortic valve and the surrounding vascular and cardiac structures.

Operative Considerations

Cardiac catheterization is recommended for children with aortic stenosis when they become symptomatic or develop electrocardiographic changes. Aortic valvotomy is indicated for patients with significant symptoms or those whose catheterization data indicate moderate or severe stenosis. In children, the stenotic valve is pliable enough for valvotomy so that an aortic valve prosthesis is not required. Ultimately, children who have undergone aortic valvotomy may require a prosthesis in adulthood if the valve becomes calcified, rigid, or stenotic.

Summary

In aortic valvular stenosis, a suprasternal notch thrill is present, associated with an ejection type murmur in the aortic area and an aortic ejection click. X-ray examination may show cardiomegaly, but is usually normal. The electrocardiogram is the most crucial laboratory examination in following the course of the patient. The electrocardiographic findings of left ventricular strain or chest pain or syncope alert the physician that further diagnostic studies and surgery should be performed.

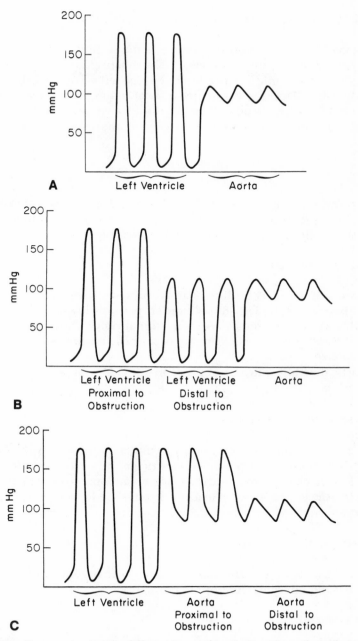

Figure 30. Pressure tracings in different types of aortic stenosis as the catheter is withdrawn from the left ventricle to the aorta. A. Valvular aortic stenosis. B. Subvalvular aortic stenosis. C. Supravalvular aortic stenosis.

DISCRETE MEMBRANOUS SUBAORTIC STENOSIS

Discrete membranous subaortic stenosis is the second most common form of left ventricular outflow obstruction. This obstruction is a fibrous membrane with a small central orifice located in the left ventricle within 1 cm of the aortic valve. Through the orifice a jet of blood passes and strikes the aortic valve. Because the jet strikes the aortic valve, the energy of the jet is dissipated so that poststenotic dilatation of the ascending aorta rarely occurs.

History

The murmur is usually recognized in infancy. Congestive cardiac failure is rare. The symptoms of chest pain and syncope may occur in patients with severe obstruction, but most patients are asymptomatic.

Physical Examination

The prominent physical finding is an aortic systolic ejection murmur that is heard best along the left sternal border, perhaps lower than in patients with valvular aortic stenosis. A suprasternal notch thrill is infrequently present. Systolic ejection clicks rarely occur because the ascending aorta is of normal size.

An aortic diastolic murmur of aortic insufficiency is present in about 70 percent of the patients.

Electrocardiographic Features

The electrocardiogram shows findings similar to those of valvular aortic stenosis. As might be expected, left ventricular hypertrophy is found, and ST and T wave changes may indicate ischemia. Some patients have an rSr' pattern in lead V_1 and an Rs in lead V_6. The reason for the latter findings is unknown.

Roentgenographic Features

The size of the heart is normal and there is no enlargement of the ascending aorta. Pulmonary vasculature is normal.

Natural History

Discrete membranous subaortic stenosis is considered to be a progressive lesion, probably not because of progressive narrowing of the orifice in the membrane. There is probably progressive fibrosis of the left ventricle secondary to inability to supply the increased oxygen demands of the left ventricle. The aortic insufficiency develops and progresses probably secondary to the trauma of the jet upon the aortic valve.

Cardiac Catheterization

Oxygen data are normal. A systolic pressure gradient is found below the level of the aortic valve within the left ventricle (Fig. 30). Angiography is indicated to identify the location of the membrane. If aortic insufficiency is present, it is best observed following aortography; otherwise, left ventriculography is indicated.

Operative Considerations

Excision of the membrane is indicated in almost all patients in whom it is found, unless a small gradient is found at cardiac catheterization. The purposes of operation are relief of the elevated left ventricular systolic pressure and reduction of the trauma to the aortic valve.

Postoperative Results

The operative risk is low and approaches that of valvular aortic stenosis. The results are usually very good, with the left ventricular systolic pressure approaching normal postoperatively. Following operation, the degree of aortic insufficiency is usually less. The major hazard of the operation is the possibility of damage to the septal leaflet of the mitral valve, since the membrane is attached to this leaflet.

Summary

Discrete membranous subaortic stenosis clinically resembles valvular aortic stenosis in many respects, but it lacks the clinical and roentgenographic findings of poststenotic dilatation of the aorta.

SUPRAVALVULAR AORTIC STENOSIS

Obstruction to left ventricular outflow can also result from supravalvular stenosis. In most patients, the ascending aorta narrows in an hourglass deformity. Although the defect is usually limited to the ascending aorta, other arteries, such as the brachiocephalic and, infrequently, the renal arteries may also be narrowed. Peripheral pulmonary arterial stenosis may coexist.

In this form of aortic stenosis the systolic pressure is elevated in the ascending aorta proximal to the obstruction, and the coronary arteries are submitted to an elevated systolic pressure. The elevation can lead to tortuosity of the coronary arteries and premature atherosclerosis.

Two factors have been implicated in the etiology of this condition. The first is infantile idiopathic hypercalcemia. A few patients with idiopathic hypercalcemia in infancy have subsequently been diagnosed as having supravalvular aortic stenosis. Other children with supravalvular aortic stenosis, but without documented hypercalcemia in infancy, have a facial appearance similar to that of children with idiopathic hypercalcemia. Secondly, supravalvular aortic stenosis also shows a strong familial tendency.

History

Most of our patients have been asymptomatic; cardiac disease has been identified by the presence of a murmur or by the facial characteristics associated with idiopathic hypercalcemia. Congestive cardiac failure or growth retardation is rare as in other forms of aortic stenosis, but sudden death can occur, and perhaps the risk is higher because of acquired abnormalities of the coronary arteries.

Physical Examination

The general physical characteristics of the child, particularly the facies, may suggest the diagnosis of supravalvular aortic stenosis. The facies, described as elfinlike, are characterized by puffy upper eyelids and prominent epicanthal folds, long upper lip, and cupid-bow mouth. The development and growth of the child with abnormal facies may be mildly retarded. The cry or voice has a typical brassy quality. Many other children have a normal appearance.

Supravalvular aortic stenosis can be suspected by careful blood pressure recording in both arms and legs. A blood pressure discrepancy between the arms of at least 20 mm Hg is found. This is related to a narrowing of a subclavian artery or to the pressure effect of the jet into the origin of the right subclavian artery.

An aortic systolic ejection murmur is the prominent cardiac finding, and in contrast to valvular stenosis is located maximally beneath the right clavicle and not along the left sternal border. A systolic ejection click is *not* present because there is no poststenotic dilatation. Diastole is clear.

Electrocardiographic Features

The electrocardiogram usually shows features similar to those of valvular aortic stenosis, and would be expected to show left ventricular hypertrophy. Some patients, for unknown reasons, show an rSr' pattern in lead V_1 and an Rs in lead V_6, and no voltage criteria of left ventricular hypertrophy. The ST segment and T wave changes may be present, reflecting myocardial ischemia that may be accentuated by coronary arterial abnormalities.

Roentgenographic Features

The cardiac size is normal and poststenotic dilatation is absent.

Natural History

The major change believed to occur during the course of this disease is the development of myocardial ischemia and fibrosis, and its consequences. Therefore, in following the patient, attention must be directed to the history of syncope or chest pain and to electrocardiographic changes in the ST segment and T waves.

Cardiac Catheterization

The oxygen data are normal. The diagnosis is established by measuring a systolic pressure difference in the ascending aorta (Fig. 30). Angiography can demonstrate the anatomic details of the obstruction and can identify associated lesions, such as coexistent peripheral pulmonary arterial stenosis.

Operative Considerations

Operative relief of the obstruction is indicated if the obstruction leads to a gradient of more than 30 or 40 mm Hg, or if there are symptoms related to myocardial ischemia. A longitudinal incision is made across the stenotic area, and the area is widened by placement of a diamond-shaped patch. During the operation, the coronary ostia are explored to make certain they are patent. Occasionally, coronary arterial bypass is indicated.

Postoperative Results

The operative risk for supravalvular aortic stenosis is higher than for valvular aortic stenosis. Long-term follow-up data are not available.

Summary

Supravalvular aortic stenosis differs from valvular aortic stenosis, since findings of poststenotic dilatation are absent. Characteristic facies are seen in some patients.

Pulmonary Stenosis

Pulmonary stenosis (Fig. 31) can occur at three sites in the outflow area of the right side of the heart: below the pulmonary valve (infundibular), at the level of the valve (valvular), or above the valve (supravalvular). Infundibular pulmonary stenosis rarely occurs as an isolated lesion. Supravalvular stenosis or stenosis of the individual pulmonary arteries is also uncommon. In the majority of patients, obstruction occurs at the level of the pulmonary valve.

Regardless of the anatomic type of stenosis, the results are similar. Blood flow through the stenotic area is turbulent and leads to murmurs. The other major effect is an increase in right ventricular systolic pressure. This is illustrated best by the formula used to calculate the area of the stenotic pulmonary valve orifice in pulmonary stenosis:

$$PVA = \frac{\dfrac{\text{Cardiac Output}}{\text{SEP} \times \text{HR}}}{K \sqrt{\text{RVSP} - \text{PA}}}$$

PVA = pulmonary valve area (orifice size)
RVSP = mean right ventricular systolic pressure
PA = mean pulmonary arterial pressure
K = constant
SEP = systolic ejection period
HR = heart rate

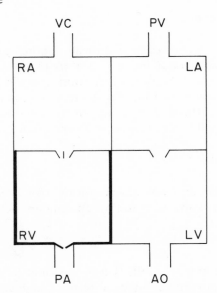

Figure 31. Central circulation in valvular pulmonary stenosis.

104

Because of the restricted orifice, the level of right ventricular systolic pressure increases to maintain a normal cardiac output. With the elevation of right ventricular systolic pressure, right ventricular hypertrophy develops, the degree paralleling the level of pressure elevation. As a consequence of the hypertrophy, right ventricular compliance can be reduced, elevating right atrial pressure and causing right atrial enlargement. As a result of the right atrial changes, the foramen ovale may be stretched open, leading to a right-to-left shunt at the atrial level. Right ventricular compliance may be reduced by the development of myocardial fibrosis, secondary to the inability to meet augmented myocardial oxygen requirements.

A second complication of right ventricular hypertrophy is the development of infundibular stenosis that may become so significant as to pose a secondary area of obstruction.

The clinical and laboratory manifestations of right ventricular hypertrophy serve as indicators of the severity of the pulmonary stenosis.

VALVULAR PULMONARY STENOSIS

In the usual form of pulmonary stenosis, the valve cusps are fused and the valve appears domed. There is a small central orifice and poststenotic dilatation.

History

There is no sex predilection in pulmonary stenosis. The murmur of pulmonary stenosis is frequently heard in the neonatal period. Many of the patients are completely asymptomatic throughout childhood, while those with more severe degrees of pulmonary stenosis may complain of fatigue on exercise. A few of the patients present with cyanosis and cardiac failure. This combination of cyanosis and failure in pulmonary stenosis with intact ventricular septum is most frequently seen in the first year of life, although it may occur at any age, and indicates severe stenosis and decompensation of the right ventricle.

Physical Examination

Most of the children appear normal, although cyanosis and clubbing exist in the few with right-to-left atrial shunt. In most patients the cardiac apex is not displaced. Typically, a systolic thrill is present below the left clavicle and upper left sternal border and, occasionally, in the suprasternal notch. An ejection type systolic murmur, heard along the upper left sternal border and below the clavicle, is transmitted to the left upper back. Usually the murmurs are loud (grade IV/VI) because the volume of flow across the valve is normal, but in patients with severe stenosis, particularly with cyanosis or cardiac failure, the murmur may be soft. The quality and characteristics of the second heart sound may also give an indication of the severity of the stenosis. In severe stenosis the pulmonary valve closure sound is delayed and soft; i.e., it may be so soft that the second heart sound appears single. A pulmonary systolic ejection click may initiate the murmur, and indicates poststenotic dilatation of the pulmonary artery. This finding is almost always present in mild to moderate pulmonary stenosis, but it may be absent in severe pulmonary stenosis.

Electrocardiographic Features

The electrocardiogram is useful in estimating the severity of the pulmonary stenosis. In mild pulmonary stenosis the electrocardiogram may be normal. With more severe degrees of stenosis, right axis deviation and right ventricular hypertrophy are present, with a tall R wave in lead V_1 and a prominent S wave in lead V_6. The height of the R wave roughly correlates with the level of right ventricular systolic pressure. Right atrial enlargement is commonly present and reflects elevated right ventricular filling pressure. In patients with severe stenosis, a pattern of right ventricular strain may develop that is manifested by deep inversion of T waves of the right precordial leads and accompanied by ST segment depression. Inverted T waves in leads V_1 to V_4 in themselves do not indicate strain because in children of most ages such a pattern is normal.

Roentgenographic Features

Usually the heart size is normal, because the right heart volume is usually normal. Patients with congestive cardiac failure or cyanosis show cardiac enlargement because of increased volume in the right atrium and right ventricle.

Except in patients with cyanosis, the pulmonary vascularity appears normal, not decreased, because in most patients with pulmonary stenosis the systemic output is normal; therefore, a normal quantity of blood must pass through the pulmonary valve.

A distinctive feature of pulmonary valvular stenosis is poststenotic dilatation of the pulmonary trunk and the left pulmonary artery (Fig. 32). This appears as a prominent bulge along the upper left cardiac border. In patients with severe stenosis, this finding may be absent.

Summary of Clinical Findings

The systolic ejection murmur indicates the turbulence of flow through the stenotic pulmonary valve. Poststenotic dilatation is indicated by the

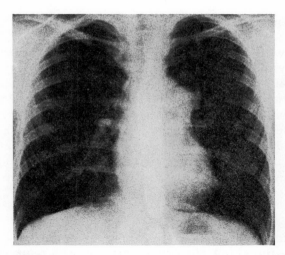

Figure 32. Thoracic roentgenogram in pulmonary stenosis. Normal-sized heart and pulmonary vasculature. Poststenotic dilatation of pulmonary artery.

pulmonary systolic ejection click and the roentgenographic findings of an enlarged pulmonary trunk. The electrocardiogram is the best indicator of the degree of right ventricular hypertrophy. Right atrial enlargement, cyanosis, and congestive cardiac failure are indicators of altered right ventricular compliance from severe right ventricular hypertrophy and/or fibrosis.

Natural History

The orifice of the stenotic pulmonary valve increases as the child grows, so that the degree of obstruction does not increase with age. The deterioration of the clinical status that occurs in some patients appears to result from altered right ventricular myocardial performance related to fibrosis. This complication occurs in infancy and in adulthood, but rarely in the mid-childhood years.

Cardiac Catheterization

Oximetry data are normal except in the occasional patient with a right-to-left shunt at the atrial level. The right ventricular systolic pressure is elevated, while pulmonary arterial pressure is normal or low. Both the pressure data and the cardiac output data are needed to accurately assess the severity of the stenosis by calculating the pulmonary valve area. Right ventricular angiography is indicated to outline the details of the pulmonary valve and associated infundibular narrowing.

Operative Considerations

Any patient with dome-shaped pulmonary valvular stenosis and a right ventricular systolic pressure greater than 75 mm Hg should undergo a pulmonary valvotomy. This procedure carries a low risk and at some centers can be performed without the use of cardiopulmonary bypass. The results are almost always favorable, with reduction of right ventricular systolic pressure to less than 75 mm Hg. Pulmonary valvular insufficiency regularly results from valvotomy but is well tolerated because pulmonary arterial pressure is low. Infundibular narrowing does not require excision, but will regress with time if the valve is adequately opened.

Summary

Pulmonary stenosis can usually be diagnosed on the basis of clinical and laboratory findings, but cardiac catheterization is required to precisely determine the severity. Pulmonary valvotomy is indicated in patients with moderate or severe stenosis, and can be performed at low risk and with excellent results.

PULMONARY STENOSIS SECONDARY TO DYSPLASTIC PULMONARY VALVE

A distinctive form of pulmonary stenosis accounts for 10 percent of all instances of valvular pulmonary stenosis. Anatomically the pulmonary valve leaflets do not show commissural fusion as in most examples of stenotic valves. Rather, the commissures are open but each leaflet is greatly thickened and redundant. The valvular obstruction is caused by the bulk of valvular tissue located in the pulmonary annulus. The pulmonary annulus may be reduced in diameter. Poststenotic dilatation usually does not occur.

History

The history is similar to that of patients with pulmonary stenosis secondary to a dome-shaped pulmonary valve.

Physical Examination

In most patients, dysplastic pulmonary valve is associated with various noncardiac abnormalities of either the leopard or the Noonan syndromes. In the former, the general features include multiple lentigines, ocular hypertelorism, ptosis, neurosensory deafness, retarded growth, and delayed development. The Noonan syndrome has been termed male

Turner's syndrome because the phenotypic features may be similar, including webbed neck, but pulmonary stenosis is present. Chromosome studies are normal. Both of these syndromes include a small stature and show a familial tendency.

Auscultation shows a pulmonary systolic ejection murmur, usually grade II-IV/VI. Since poststenotic dilatation is not present, a systolic ejection click is not heard. The P_2 may be soft and delayed.

Electrocardiographic Features

The electrocardiogram is distinctive. The QRS axis is almost always superiorly directed ($-60°$ to $-150°$) and distinguishes the dysplastic valve from dome-shaped pulmonary stenosis, in which the QRS axis rarely exceeds $+180°$. The reason for this alteration of the QRS axis is unknown, but perhaps it represents an abnormality in the location of the conduction system.

Right ventricular hypertrophy is present, the degree reflecting the level of right ventricular systolic pressure. Right atrial enlargement may be present.

Roentgenographic Features

The heart size is normal, as is the vascularity. The pulmonary arterial segment is normal size as compared to dome-shaped pulmonary stenosis.

Natural History

In this form of pulmonary stenosis the stenotic valve orifice probably grows in relation to the growth of the child. Changes that may occur with age are related to the effect of the elevated right ventricular systolic pressure and right ventricular hypertrophy upon the right ventricle.

Cardiac Catheterization

The data obtained at cardiac catheterization are similar to that obtained in dome-shaped pulmonary stenosis. However, angiography confirms the dysplastic nature of the valve because the valve leaflets appear thickened and immobile. The pulmonary artery is slightly enlarged.

Operative Considerations

The indications for operation are similar to those of dome-shaped pulmonary stenosis; the operative approach, however, is different. Valvotomy cannot be performed because commissural fusion is not present.

One or two leaflets must be excised, and in some patients a patch must be placed across the annulus to widen this area of right ventricular outflow.

PERIPHERAL PULMONARY ARTERY STENOSIS

Stenosis can occur above the pulmonary valve and in the branches of the pulmonary arteries. One or more major branches may be involved, showing either a long area of narrowing or a discrete narrowing. In the other examples, the entire pulmonary arterial tree may be hypoplastic.

Peripheral pulmonary artery stenosis can result from the congenital rubella syndrome; can occur in children with supravalvular aortic stenosis; or can occur without apparent cause.

History

Most patients with this condition are asymptomatic.

Physical Examination

There may be features of congenital rubella syndrome or supravalvular aortic stenosis. Occasionally normal newborn infants have auscultatory findings of peripheral pulmonary artery stenosis, but the findings may disappear with time.

The classic finding is a systolic ejection type murmur present under the left clavicle and heard well throughout both the lung fields and the axillae. The second heart sound is normal, and a systolic ejection click is not heard because the pulmonary artery is not dilated, but it may be small.

Electrocardiographic Features

There are no features distinguishing peripheral pulmonary artery stenosis from valvular pulmonary stenosis. It shows right ventricular hypertrophy proportional to the degree of hypertrophy.

Roentgenographic Features

The x-rays are usually normal.

Natural History

The degree of stenosis does not increase with age; it has been considered a benign condition since the degree of obstruction is usually mild.

Cardiac Catheterization

Oxygen data are normal. Pressure tracings show a systolic gradient in the pulmonary arteries. The anatomic details are shown by pulmonary arteriography.

Operative Considerations

Most patients do not require operation as the degree of stenosis is not severe. In patients with severe obstruction, operation often cannot be performed because anatomic features such as diffuse hypoplasia of the pulmonary arteries or multiple areas of stenosis preclude an operative approach.

Summary of Obstructive Lesions (Table 9)

In each of the conditions discussed, turbulence occurs through a narrowed orifice, causing a systolic ejection murmur. Beyond the obstruction, post-stenotic dilatation occurs; this can be evidenced either by roentgenographic findings or by an ejection click. The restricted orifice leads to elevation of systolic pressures proximally, and to ventricular hypertrophy. The clinical and laboratory findings reflecting this hypertrophy permit assessment of the severity of the condition.

CARDIAC CONDITIONS ASSOCIATED WITH RIGHT-TO-LEFT SHUNT

In most patients with cyanosis related to congenital cardiac abnormalities, an abnormality is present that permits a portion of the systemic venous return to bypass the lungs and to enter the systemic circulation directly. Right-to-left shunt results from two general types of cardiac malformations: conditions that permit admixture of the systemic and pulmonary venous returns, and conditions with obstruction to pulmonary blood flow and an intracardiac defect. The first group shows increased pulmonary vascularity, and the second shows diminished pulmonary vascularity. The most common conditions resulting in cyanosis may be divided between the following two categories.

    Admixture lesions (increased pulmonary vascularity):
        Complete transposition of the great arteries
        Total anomalous pulmonary venous connection
        Persistent truncus arteriosus
    Cyanosis and diminished blood flow:
        Tetralogy of Fallot
        Tricuspid atresia
        Pulmonary atresia
        Ebstein's malformation

Regardless of the type of cardiac malformation leading to cyanosis, polycythemia, clubbing, slow growth, and a risk of brain abscess are associated. The first three findings are related to tissue hypoxia and have been discussed previously. Brain abscess is probably a result of bacteria

TABLE 9. SUMMARY OF OBSTRUCTIVE LESIONS

Malformation		HISTORY					PHYSICAL EXAMINATION		
	Sex	Major Syndrome	Age Murmur	Congestive Cardiac Failure	Symptoms	Blood Pressure	Thrill	Murmur	Ejection Click
Coarctation of aorta	M > F	Turner	Infancy	±	Headache	Diminished in legs	Suprasternal notch	Systolic—precordial and back	Aortic (if bicuspid valve)
Aortic stenosis	M > F	None	Birth	±	Chest pain	Normal or narrow pulse pressure	Suprasternal notch Aortic area	Ejection systolic—aortic and left sternal border	Aortic
Pulmonary stenosis	M = F	None	Birth	±	Occasional cyanosis	Normal	Suprasternal notch Pulmonic area	Ejection systolic—pulmonic area and left back	Pulmonic

| | ELECTROCARDIOGRAM | | | | ROENTGENOGRAM | | | |
Malformation	Axis	Atrial Enlargement	Ventricular Hypertrophy	Other	Aortic Enlargement	Pulmonary Artery Enlargement	Chamber Hypertrophy	Other
Coarctation of aorta	Normal	None or left	Right (infant) Left (older child)	Strain pattern if severe	Absent unless bicuspid valve	Absent	Left ventricle	Poststenotic dilatation descending aorta
Aortic stenosis	Normal	None or left	Left	Strain pattern if severe	Present	Absent	Left ventricle	None
Pulmonary stenosis	Normal or right	Normal or right	Right	Strain pattern if severe	Absent	Present	Right ventricle	None

F = female
M = male

> = greater than
± = may be present or absent

113

having direct access to the systemic circuit because of the right-to-left shunt.

Admixture Lesions

The combination of cyanosis and increased pulmonary vascular markings indicates an admixture lesion. In most cardiac malformations classified in this group, a single chamber receives the total systemic and pulmonary venous returns. The admixture lesion can occur at any cardiac level: venous—total anomalous pulmonary venous connection; atrial—single atrium; ventricular—single ventricle; and great vessel—persistent truncus arteriosus. Near uniform mixing of the two venous returns usually occurs.

The hemodynamics of the admixture lesions resemble those of the left-to-right shunts occurring at the same level. The direction and magnitude of blood flow in total anomalous pulmonary venous connection and single atrium are governed as an isolated atrial septal defect by the relative ventricular compliances. Relative resistances to systemic and pulmonary flow control the distribution of blood in patients with single ventricle and persistent truncus arteriosus in a way similar to the case in ventricular septal defect. Thus, the natural history and many of the clinical and laboratory findings of the admixture lesions are identical to those of left-to-right shunts, including the development of pulmonary vascular disease.

In admixture lesions the systemic arterial oxygen saturation or the hemoglobin and hematocrit values are valuable indicators of the volume of pulmonary blood flow, as the degree of cyanosis is inversely related to the volume of pulmonary blood flow. In patients with large pulmonary blood flow the degree of cyanosis is slight, since large amounts of fully saturated blood return from the lungs and mix with a relatively smaller volume of systemic venous return. Should the patient develop pulmonary vascular disease or another factor that limits pulmonary blood flow, the amount of fully oxygenated blood returning from the lung and mixing with the systemic venous return is reduced, so the patient becomes more cyanotic and his hemoglobin and hematocrit values rise.

Complete transposition is included in the admixture group because the patients are cyanotic and have increased pulmonary blood flow. They usually have only partial admixture of the two venous returns; this incomplete mixing leads to symptoms of severe hypoxia.

COMPLETE TRANSPOSITION OF THE GREAT ARTERIES

The term *transposition* indicates an anatomic reversal in anteroposterior relationships. Since normally the pulmonary artery lies anterior to the aorta, in complete transposition of the great arteries (Fig. 33) the aorta lies anteriorly to the pulmonary artery. While normally the anterior blood vessel arises from the infundibulum, which is the conus portion of the right ventricle, the aorta in complete transposition arises from the right ventricle. The pulmonary trunk, on the other hand, originates from the left ventricle. Because of the transposition of the great vessels and their anomalous anatomic relationship to the ventricles, two more or less independent circulations exist. The systemic venous blood returns to the right atrium, enters the right ventricle, and is ejected into the aorta, while the pulmonary venous blood flows through the left side of the heart into the pulmonary artery and returns to the lungs.

A communication must exist between the left and right sides of the heart to allow some mixing of the pulmonary and systemic venous returns. The communication may be any one of the following: patent foramen ovale, atrial septal defect, ventricular septal defect, or patent ductus arteriosus. In half of the patients the ventricular septum is intact and the shunt occurs at the atrial level. In the other half a ventricular septal defect is present. Pulmonary stenosis may coexist.

In patients with an intact ventricular septum, the communication, either a patent foramen ovale or a patent ductus arteriosus, between the two sides of the circulation is often narrow. As these communications follow a normal neonatal course of closing, the patients with an intact septum develop profound cyanosis in the neonatal period. A greater degree of mixing usually occurs in patients with a coexistent ventricular septal defect.

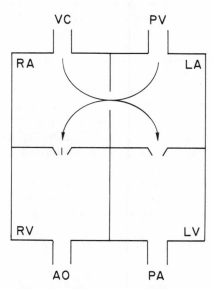

Figure 33. Central circulation in complete transposition of the great vessels.

History

Complete transposition of the great arteries occurs more frequently in male infants. Cyanosis becomes evident shortly after birth. Almost all infants exhibit dyspnea and other signs of cardiac failure in the first month of life. Infants with intact ventricular septum develop cardiac symptoms earlier and are more intensely cyanotic than those with co-existent ventricular septal defect. In the absence of operative relief, death occurs in almost every patient by 6 months of age. Patients with ventricular septal defect and pulmonary stenosis are often the least symptomatic because the pulmonary stenosis prevents excessive pulmonary blood flow and enhances flow of fully saturated blood through the ventricular septal defect into the aorta; these patients resemble those with tetralogy of Fallot.

Physical Examination

Aside from cyanosis and congestive cardiac failure, the physical findings vary, depending upon the defect associated with complete transposition of the great vessels.

With an intact ventricular septum, the intracardiac shunt is usually at the atrial level. In these cases, either no murmur is present or a soft, nonspecific murmur is audible. With an associated ventricular septal defect, a louder murmur is present. The second heart sound appears single and loud along the upper left sternal border, representing closure of the anteriorly placed aortic valve. Thus, the murmur is not helpful in diagnosing transposition of the great vessels, although it may indicate the type of associated defect. If pulmonary stenosis coexists, the murmur often radiates to the right side of the back.

Electrocardiographic Features

Since the aorta arises from the right ventricle, the pressure in the right ventricle is elevated to systemic levels and is associated with a thick-walled right ventricle. The electrocardiogram reflects this by a pattern of right axis deviation and right ventricular hypertrophy. The latter is manifested by tall R waves in the right precordial leads. Right atrial enlargement may also be observed.

Patients with a large volume of pulmonary blood flow, as with co-existent ventricular septal defect, may also exhibit left ventricular hypertrophy because of the volume load on the left ventricle.

Roentgenographic Features

Cardiomegaly is almost always present. The cardiac silhouette has a characteristic egg-shaped appearance (Fig. 34), and the superior mediastinum is narrow because the great vessels lie one in front of the other and the thymus is unusually small. Left atrial enlargement is present in the unoperated patient.

Summary of Clinical Findings

The diagnosis of complete transposition is usually indicated by a combination of rather intense cyanosis in the neonatal period, roentgenographic findings of increased pulmonary vasculature, and characteristic cardiac contour.

Cardiac Catheterization

In patients with an intact septum, oximetry data show little increase in oxygen saturation values through the right side of the heart, and little decrease in oxygen saturation is found through the left side of the heart. Among those with coexistent ventricular septal defect, larger changes in oxygen values are found. The oxygen saturation values in the pulmonary artery are higher than in the aorta, a finding virtually diagnostic of transposition of the great vessels.

In all patients the right ventricular systolic pressure is elevated. When the ventricular septum is intact, left ventricular pressure is low, but in most patients with coexistent ventricular septal defect the pressure is elevated to levels similar to those of the right ventricle.

Angiography confirms the diagnosis by showing the aorta arising from the right ventricle (Fig. 35) and the pulmonary artery arising from the left ventricle, and identifies the type of coexistent malformation.

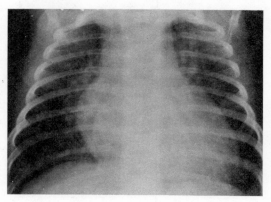

Figure 34. Thoracic roentgenogram in complete transposition of the great vessels: cardiomegaly, narrow mediastinum, increased pulmonary vasculature.

Operative Considerations

Hypoxia, one of the major symptoms of infants with transposition of the great vessels, results from inadequate mixing of the two venous returns. All patients with complete transposition of the great arteries and inadequate mixing benefit from the creation of an atrial septal defect.

At cardiac catheterization, the atrial communication can be enlarged by the Rashkind procedure. A balloon type catheter is advanced into the left atrium through the foramen ovale. The balloon is inflated and rapidly and forcefully withdrawn across the septum, tearing a larger defect and often improving the hypoxia.

If the procedure is unsuccessful in relieving the symptoms of hypoxia, a Blalock-Hanlon procedure is indicated. In this procedure an atrial septal defect is created operatively without the use of cardiopulmonary bypass. If the ventricular septal defect coexists, pulmonary arterial banding can also be performed to prevent the rapid development of pulmonary vascular disease that occurs in such patients. At some centers, patients with coexistent ventricular septal defect are not submitted to pulmonary arterial banding, but undergo a corrective operation at an early age.

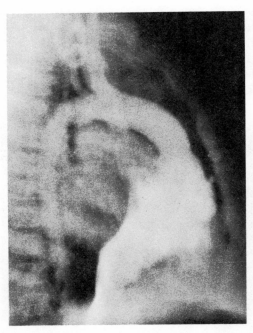

Figure 35. Venous angiogram. Lateral view. Complete transposition of the great vessels. Contrast material enters the heart through the inferior vena cava. Right ventricle and aorta opacify. Aorta located anteriorly, immediately beneath sternum.

Corrective operation is recommended by 1 year of age for most children with complete transposition of the great arteries because of the tendency to develop pulmonary vascular changes at an early age. The procedure currently used was devised by Mustard, and involves removal of the atrial septum and insertion of a pericardial baffle into the atrium to divert the systemic venous return into the left ventricle and thus to the lungs, while the pulmonary venous return is directed to the right ventricle and thus to the aorta. Although seemingly a very complicated procedure, it can be performed at a low risk in patients with intact ventricular septum but at a higher risk in patients with ventricular septal defect.

The long-term results of the Mustard procedure are not fully known. Arrhythmias are the most frequent long-term complication and are often related to abnormalities of the sinoatrial node. In addition, the venous return, either systemic or pulmonary, can be obstructed by contraction of the baffle and by constriction of the venous pathway.

Summary

Complete transposition of the great arteries is a common cardiac anomaly and results in neonatal cyanosis and cardiac failure. The physical findings and electrocardiogram vary with associated malformations. Thoracic roentgenographic studies reveal cardiomegaly and increased pulmonary vascularity. Palliative and corrective procedures are available.

TOTAL ANOMALOUS PULMONARY VENOUS CONNECTION

In total anomalous pulmonary venous connection (Fig. 36), the pulmonary veins, instead of joining the left atrium, connect with a venous channel that delivers the pulmonary venous blood to the right side of the heart. Developmentally, this anomaly results from failure of incorporation of the pulmonary veins into the left atrium, so that the pulmonary venous system retains an earlier embryologic communication to the systemic venous system.

In the embryo, the pulmonary veins communicate with both the left and right anterior cardinal veins and the umbilical vitelline system. If the pulmonary veins are not incorporated into the left atrium, pulmonary venous connection persists to one of the following structures: right superior vena cava (right anterior cardinal vein), left superior vena cava (distal left anterior cardinal vein), coronary sinus (proximal left anterior cardinal vein), or infradiaphragmatic site (umbilical-vitelline system), usually a tributary of the portal system.

Therefore, the right atrium receives not only the entire systemic venous return but also the entire pulmonary venous return. The left atrium has no direct venous supply. An obligatory right-to-left shunt exists at the atrial level through either a patent foramen ovale or an atrial septal defect.

The volume of blood shunted from the right to the left atrium and the volume of blood that enters the right ventricle are dependent upon the relative compliances of the ventricles. Ventricular compliance is influenced by ventricular pressures and vascular resistances. Right ventricular compliance normally falls following birth as a result of the normal neonatal decrease in pulmonary vascular resistance and pulmonary arterial pressure. Therefore, in most patients with total anomalous pulmonary venous connection, pulmonary blood flow is considerably greater than normal and the systemic blood flow is usually normal. Since there is a disparity between the volume of blood being carried by the right and left sides of the heart, the right side is dilated and hypertrophied, whereas the left side is relatively smaller but is usually near normal size.

In patients with total anomalous pulmonary venous connection, the degree of cyanosis is inversely related to the volume of pulmonary blood flow. The larger the volume of pulmonary blood flow, the greater the proportion of the pulmonary venous blood to total venous blood returning to the right atrium. As a result, the saturation of blood shunted to the left side of the heart may be only slightly reduced from normal. On the other hand, in hemodynamic situations in which the resistance to flow through the lungs is increased, as in the neonatal period, the volume of blood flow through the lungs is nearly normal, that is, equal to systemic blood flow. Therefore, the pulmonary and systemic venous systems in

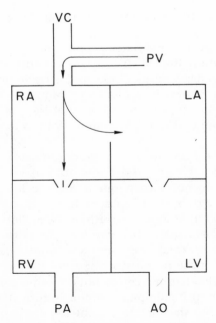

Figure 36. Central circulation in total anomalous pulmonary venous connection.

these latter situations will contribute nearly equal volumes of blood to the right atrium. The patient in these instances exhibits noticeable cyanosis.

Total anomalous pulmonary venous connection is an example of bidirectional shunting: right-to-left shunt and a left-to-right shunt at the atrial level, since all the pulmonary venous blood returns to the right atrium.

TOTAL ANOMALOUS PULMONARY VENOUS CONNECTION WITHOUT OBSTRUCTION

Total anomalous pulmonary venous connection presents two clinical pictures. One resembles atrial septal defect and the other shows intense cyanosis and a roentgenographic pattern of pulmonary venous obstruction. In the second the connecting venous channel is narrowed and obstructed, while in the first the venous channel has no obstruction.

History

The age of onset and the clinical manifestations of patients with total anomalous pulmonary venous connection vary considerably. Most patients develop congestive cardiac failure in infancy, grow slowly, and have frequent respiratory infections, but a few may be asymptomatic into later childhood.

Physical Examination

The degree of cyanosis varies as previously described because of differences in the amount of pulmonary blood flow. Most children appear acyanotic or show only slight cyanosis, although systemic arterial desaturation is always present.

The physical findings mimic isolated atrial septal defect. Cardiomegaly, precordial bulge, and right ventricular heave are found. A grade II-III/VI pulmonary systolic ejection murmur due to excess flow across the pulmonary valve is present along the upper left sternal border. Wide, fixed splitting of the second heart sound is present, and the pulmonary component may be accentuated, reflecting pulmonary hypertension. A diastolic murmur due to increased blood flow across the tricuspid valve is present along the lower left sternal border and is associated with greatly increased pulmonary blood flow. In total anomalous pulmonary venous connection to the superior vena cava, a venous hum may be present along the upper right sternal border.

Electrocardiographic Features

The electrocardiogram reveals enlargement of the right-sided cardiac chambers by a pattern of right axis deviation, right atrial enlargement, and right ventricular hypertrophy. The pattern of right ventricular hypertrophy is usually of the type reflecting volume overload—an rSR' pattern in lead V_1.

Roentgenographic Features

The roentgenographic findings also resemble isolated atrial septal defect. Cardiomegaly, primarily of right-sided chambers, and increased pulmonary blood flow are found on the roentgenogram. In contrast to most other admixture lesions, the left atrium is not enlarged, because blood flow through this chamber is normal.

Except for total anomalous pulmonary venous connection of the left superior vena cava, the roentgenographic contour is not characteristic. In this form the cardiac silhouette has been described as a figure eight or "snowman heart" (Fig. 37). The upper portion of the cardiac contour is formed by the left and right superior venae cavae, which are enlarged since they both are carrying the pulmonary venous return. The lower portion of the contour is formed by the bulk of the heart.

Summary of Clinical Findings

The clinical, electrocardiographic, and roentgenographic findings of total anomalous pulmonary venous connection, without obstruction to pulmonary blood flow, resemble those of atrial septal defect because the effects upon the heart are similar. Cyanosis should serve to distinguish the conditions, although it may be minimal or not clinically evident. Unlike the case in uncomplicated atrial septal defect, congestive cardiac failure and elevated pulmonary arterial pressure may be found in total anomalous pulmonary venous connection.

Cardiac Catheterization

The oxygen saturation values in each cardiac chamber and in both great vessels are virtually identical. An increase in oxygen saturation may be found in the vena cava, coronary sinus, or other venous sites into which the pulmonary venous blood flows. The saturation of blood in the left atrium and left ventricle is reduced because of the obligatory right-to-left atrial shunt.

Pulmonary hypertension may be found in infants, but some patients, particularly older ones, show near-normal levels of pulmonary arterial pressures.

Pulmonary angiography is indicated in these patients. During the later phases of the study, the pulmonary veins opacify and subsequently fill the connecting venous channel. This serves to identify the anatomic form of anomalous pulmonary venous connection.

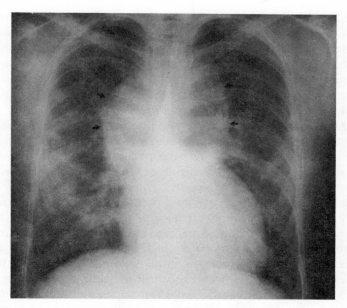

Figure 37. Thoracic roentgenogram. AP view. Total anomalous pulmonary venous connection to left superior vena cava, yielding snowman heart. Upper portion of cardiac silhouette (arrows) formed by dilated right and left superior venae cavae.

Operative Considerations

Under cardiopulmonary bypass, the confluence of pulmonary veins is connected to the left atrium. At the same time, the atrial communication is closed and the connecting vessel is divided. In many older infants and children, this operation can be performed at a low risk, but in neonates and younger infants, the risk remains high.

Summary

Each of the anatomic types of total anomalous pulmonary venous connection is associated with cyanosis of variable degree. The physical findings are those of atrial septal defect, and findings of pulmonary hypertension may also be found. Both the electrocardiogram and the thoracic roentgenogram reveal enlargement of the right-sided cardiac chambers. Corrective operations can be performed successfully for each of the forms of total anomalous pulmonary venous connection.

TOTAL ANOMALOUS PULMONARY VENOUS CONNECTION WITH OBSTRUCTION

In total anomalous pulmonary venous connection, an obstruction can be present in the channel returning pulmonary venous blood to the right side of the heart. This is always true in patients with an infradiaphragmatic connection and occasionally in patients with a supradiaphragmatic connection. In the latter, obstruction may occur intrinsically from narrowing of the channel or extrinsically as the channel passes between the bronchus and the pulmonary artery. In infradiaphragmatic connection, four mechanisms are responsible for obstruction in pulmonary venous flow: 1) the venous channel is long; 2) the channel traverses the diaphragm through the esophageal hiatus and can be compressed by either esophageal or diaphragmatic action; 3) the channel narrows at its junction with the portal venous system; and 4) the pulmonary venous blood must traverse the hepatic capillary system before returning to the right atrium by way of the hepatic veins.

The obstruction leads to an elevated pulmonary venous pressure. Consequently, pulmonary capillary pressure is raised, and this leads to pulmonary edema and a dilated pulmonary lymphatic system that helps remove the pulmonary edema. Pulmonary arterial pressure is also elevated, because of both elevated pulmonary capillary pressure and reflex pulmonary vasoconstriction. As a result of the pulmonary hypertension, the right ventricle remains thick-walled and does not undergo the normal evolution following birth. The right ventricle, therefore, remains relatively noncompliant, and as a result the volume of flow into the right ventricle is limited. Because of the relatively reduced pulmonary blood flow, the patient shows more intense cyanosis than patients with total anomalous pulmonary venous connection without obstruction.

The clinical features of total anomalous pulmonary venous connection with obstruction relate to the consequences of pulmonary venous obstruction and the limited pulmonary blood flow.

History

Patients with total anomalous pulmonary venous connection with obstruction in the neonatal period present cyanosis and respiratory distress. Cyanosis is often intense because the volume of pulmonary flow is quite limited due to the obstruction in the venous channel and the effect of pulmonary hypertension on reducing right ventricular compliance. The cyanosis is accentuated by the pulmonary edema that interferes with oxygen transport from the alveolus to the pulmonary capillary. Respiratory symptoms of tachypnea and dyspnea are caused by the altered compliance of the lungs produced by pulmonary edema and hypertensive pulmonary arteries.

Physical Examination

Cyanosis is present. Increased respiratory effort is manifested by intercostal retractions and tachypnea. On clinical examination the heart size is normal. In total anomalous venous connection the systolic and diastolic murmurs originate from increased blood flow across the tricuspid and pulmonary valves, respectively. In patients with obstruction to pulmonary venous flow, however, the volume of flow through the right side of the heart is normal, so that no murmurs are found. The pulmonic component of the second heart sound is accentuated, reflecting pulmonary hypertension.

Beyond the immediate neonatal period, the infant appears scrawny and malnourished.

Electrocardiographic Features

As expected, with the hemodynamics leading to right ventricular hypertrophy, right axis deviation, right atrial enlargement, and right ventricular hypertrophy are found. In a normal neonate, however, the QRS axis is normally directed toward the right, the P waves may approach 3 mm in amplitude, and the R waves are tall in the right precordial leads. Therefore, the electrocardiogram of neonates with total anomalous pulmonary venous connection may be interpreted as normal for age. Such a pattern, however, is compatible with the diagnosis.

Roentgenographic Features

Cardiac size is normal because the volume of systemic and pulmonary blood flows are normal. The pulmonary vasculature shows a diffuse reticular pattern of pulmonary edema. Even in young children, Kerley B lines, small horizontal lines at the margins of the lower lung fields, are present. The roentgenographic pattern, although similar to that of hyaline membrane disease, differs in that it does not show air bronchiograms.

Summary of Clinical Findings

This form of total anomalous pulmonary venous connection is very difficult to distinguish from neonatal pulmonary disease as the clinical and laboratory findings are similar. The patients present with respiratory distress and cyanosis in the neonatal period. No murmurs are present. The electrocardiogram may be normal for age, and the roentgenogram may show a normal-sized heart and a diffuse, hazy pattern. Often only cardiac catheterization and angiography can distinguish pulmonary disease from this form of cardiac disease.

Cardiac Catheterization

As in the form without obstruction, the oxygen saturations are identical in each cardiac chamber, but in this case the oxygen saturations are extremely low. Pulmonary hypertension is present, and the pulmonary wedge pressure is elevated as well. Angiography shows the anomalous pulmonary venous connection, which is usually connected to an infradiaphragmatic site.

Operative Considerations

Infants with total anomalous pulmonary venous connection to an infradiaphragmatic site often die in the neonatal period. Operation is indicated as soon as the diagnosis is made. The technique is as described previously.

SUMMARY

Total anomalous pulmonary venous connection, although of several anatomic forms, presents one of two clinical pictures. In one, the pulmonary arterial pressures and right ventricular compliance are normal or slightly elevated. These patients present features resembling atrial septal defect but show mild cyanosis. In the second, pulmonary arterial pressure and pulmonary resistance are elevated because of pulmonary venous obstruction. Therefore, right ventricular compliance is reduced and pulmonary blood flow is limited. These patients show a roentgenographic pattern of pulmonary venous obstruction or severe cyanosis and major respiratory symptoms. The clinical and laboratory findings resemble neonatal respiratory distress syndrome.

PERSISTENT TRUNCUS ARTERIOSUS

In persistent truncus arteriosus (Fig. 38), a single arterial blood vessel leaves the heart and gives rise to both the pulmonary and systemic circulations. This malformation is always associated with a ventricular septal defect, through which both ventricles empty into the truncus arteriosus. Because the defect is large and the truncus arteriosus essentially originates from both ventricles, the right ventricular pressure is similar to that of the left ventricle.

The hemodynamics of persistent truncus arteriosus are similar to those of ventricular septal defect and patent ductus arteriosus because the respective volumes of systemic and pulmonary blood flow are dependent upon the relative resistance to flow into the systemic circulation and into the pulmonary circulation.

The resistance to flow through the lungs is dependent upon two factors: 1) the caliber of the pulmonary arterial branches arising from the truncus arteriosus, and 2) the pulmonary vascular resistance. Although there are anatomic differences in the size of the pulmonary arterial branches as they originate from the truncus arteriosus, ordinarily their size does not offer significant resistance to pulmonary blood flow so that pulmonary arterial pressure equals that in the truncus arteriosus. Therefore the caliber of the pulmonary arterioles is the primary determinant of pulmonary blood flow. In the newborn period when pulmonary vascular resistance is elevated, the volume of blood flow through the lungs is similar to the systemic blood flow. As the pulmonary vasculature matures, the pulmonary blood flow becomes progressively larger.

Many of the clinical and laboratory findings of truncus arteriosus are dependent upon the volume of pulmonary blood flow. Increased pulmonary blood flow leads to three effects. 1. The degree of cyanosis and the volume of pulmonary blood flow are inversely related. The degree of cyanosis lessens as pulmonary blood flow increases because of the larger quantities of fully saturated pulmonary venous return mixing with the relatively fixed systemic venous return. 2. Congestive cardiac failure develops because of left ventricular volume overload. 3. The pulse pressure is widened because during diastole the blood leaves the truncus arteriosus to enter the pulmonary arteries.

The truncal valve is usually tricuspid but may become insufficient in some patients, allowing regurgitation into the ventricle. Therefore an additional volume of stress proportional to the amount of regurgitation is placed upon the ventricles.

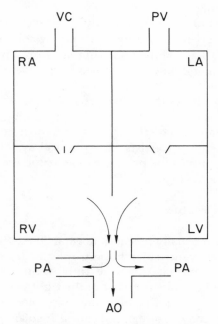

Figure 38. Central circulation in persistent truncus arteriosus.

History

The patient's symptoms vary with the volume of pulmonary blood flow. In the neonatal period, cyanosis is the major symptom because the elevated pulmonary vascular resistance limits the pulmonary blood flow. As pulmonary vascular resistance falls, cyanosis lessens, but congestive cardiac failure develops, usually after several weeks of age. Patients with truncus arteriosus and congestive cardiac failure mimic those with ventricular septal defect at this time because cyanosis may be mild or absent. Dyspnea on exertion, easy fatigability, and frequent respiratory infections are common symptoms.

Patients whose pulmonary blood flow is limited, either by the development of pulmonary vascular disease or by the presence of small pulmonary arteries arising from the truncus, show predominant symptoms related to cyanosis rather than the features of congestive cardiac failure, unless significant regurgitation through the truncal valve coexists.

Physical Examination

Cyanosis may or may not be clinically evident. Manifestations of a wide pulse pressure may be present if there is increased pulmonary blood flow or significant truncal insufficiency. Cardiomegaly and a precordial bulge are commonly present.

The auscultatory findings may initially resemble ventricular septal defect. The major auscultatory finding is a loud systolic murmur along the left sternal border. An apical diastolic rumble is present in most patients, indicating the large blood flow across the mitral valve due to the increased pulmonary blood flow.

Truncus arteriosus shows three distinctive auscultatory findings. 1. The second heart sound is single, since there is only a single semilunar valve. 2. A high pitched, early decrescendo diastolic murmur may be present if truncal valve insufficiency coexists. 3. An apical systolic ejection click is usually heard and indicates the presence of a dilated great vessel, which in this case is truncus arteriosus.

Electrocardiographic Features

The electrocardiogram usually reveals a normal QRS axis and biventricular hypertrophy. The left ventricular hypertrophy is related to the volume overload of the left ventricle, and the right ventricular hypertrophy is related to the elevated systolic pressure of the right ventricle. If pulmonary vascular disease develops, reducing pulmonary blood flow, the left ventricular hypertrophy may disappear. Truncal insufficiency, however, by augmenting the volume in either ventricle, may modify these findings.

128

Roentgenographic Features

The pulmonary vasculature is increased. There is usually a prominent "ascending aorta" representing the truncus arteriosus. Because the pulmonary arteries arise from the left side of the truncus arteriosus, a pulmonary artery segment may be present. Most patients show cardiomegaly proportionate to the volume of pulmonary blood flow and the amount of truncal insufficiency. Left atrial enlargement is found in patients with increased pulmonary blood flow. A right aortic arch is found in one quarter of the patients; this finding combined with that of increased pulmonary vascular markings and the presence of cyanosis is virtually diagnostic of truncus arteriosus.

Summary of Clinical Findings

Persistent truncus arteriosus can be suspected in a cyanotic patient who has a murmur of ventricular septal defect and two characteristic features: a single second heart sound and an early systolic ejection click. The volume of pulmonary blood flow is reflected by the degree of cyanosis and the amount of left atrial enlargement. The degree of cardiomegaly on thoracic roentgenogram or left ventricular hypertrophy on electrocardiography does not solely reflect pulmonary blood flow, since coexistent truncal insufficiency can also cause these particular findings.

Natural History

Although data are limited, the course in truncus arteriosus resembles that in ventricular septal defect. Pulmonary vascular disease occurs in these patients as in those with large ventricular septal defect, and is the ultimate threat to longevity and operability. With time, truncal insufficiency worsens.

Cardiac Catheterization

Usually the catheter can be passed into the truncus arteriosus and from there into the pulmonary arteries. The systolic pressures are identical in both ventricles and in the truncus arteriosus. A wide pulse pressure is often found in the truncus arteriosus. An increase in oxygen saturation is found in the right ventricle and further increase is found in the truncus arteriosus. The blood in the truncus arteriosus is not fully saturated.

Definitive diagnosis requires angiography into the right ventricle or truncus arteriosus. Such study also permits semiquantitation of the degree of truncal insufficiency.

Operative Considerations

For infants manifesting severe cardiac failure and for those who fail to respond to medical management, banding of the pulmonary artery can be

129

performed. Although the cardiac failure is improved and the infant grows, the band can complicate definitive repair.

In selected infants and older patients, a corrective operation is recommended. In this procedure, the ventricular septal defect is closed in such a way that left ventricular blood passes into the truncus arteriosus. The pulmonary arteries are removed and are connected to one end of a valved Dacron conduit, the other end of which is inserted into the right ventricle. If severe, truncal insufficiency can be corrected simultaneously by insertion of a prosthetic valve. The risk is considerably higher in patients with pulmonary vascular disease. A few centers have reported success in corrective surgery during infancy, although, obviously, reoperation will be necessary.

Summary

Persistent truncus arteriosus is an infrequently occurring cardiac anomaly whose clinical and laboratory features resemble ventricular septal defect and patent ductus arteriosus as the hemodynamics and natural history are similar. Corrective operations are available, but the long-term results await full evaluation.

Cyanosis and Diminished Pulmonary Blood Flow

Patients with cyanosis and roentgenographic evidence of diminished pulmonary blood flow have cardiac malformations in which there is obstruction to pulmonary blood flow and an intracardiac defect that permits a right-to-left shunt. The degree of cyanosis varies inversely with the volume of pulmonary blood flow. The volume that pulmonary blood flow is reduced equals the volume shunted in a right-to-left direction.

The intracardiac right-to-left shunt can occur at either the ventricular or the atrial level. In patients with a ventricular shunt, the cardiac size is usually normal, as in tetralogy of Fallot; whereas those with atrial shunts, such as tricuspid atresia or Ebstein's malformation, show cardiomegaly.

TETRALOGY OF FALLOT

Tetralogy of Fallot (Fig. 39) is probably the most widely known cardiac condition resulting in cyanosis. This malformation has four components: ventricular septal defect; aorta, overriding the ventricular septal defect; pulmonary stenosis, generally infundibular in location; and right ventricular hypertrophy. Because of the relationship of the aorta and right ventricle, right ventricular systolic pressure is at systemic levels.

Hemodynamically, tetralogy of Fallot can be considered a combination of large ventricular septal defect, allowing equalization of ventricular sys-

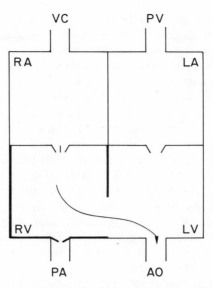

Figure 39. Central circulation in tetralogy of Fallot.

tolic pressures, and severe pulmonary stenosis, so the pulmonary arterial pressure is lower than normal. The magnitude of the shunt through the ventricular communication is dependent upon the relative resistances of the pulmonary stenosis and the systemic circulation. Because the pulmonary stenosis is frequently related to a narrowed infundibulum, it responds to catecholamines and other stimuli. Therefore, the amount of right-to-left shunt and the degree of cyanosis vary considerably with factors such as emotion and exercise. Many of the symptoms of tetralogy of Fallot are related to sudden changes in either of these resistance factors.

Tetralogy of Fallot may be associated with pulmonary valve atresia and has been called pseudotruncus arteriosus. In this anomaly, blood cannot flow directly from the right ventricle into the pulmonary artery, and the entire output from both ventricles is into the aorta. The pulmonary circulation of these patients is supplied either by bronchial arteries acting as collaterals or through a patent ductus arteriosus. Severe hypoxic symptoms may develop in the neonatal period if the patent ductus arteriosus closes or if the bronchials are narrow.

History

The children often become cyanotic in the first year of life, some in the neonatal period. The time of appearance and the severity of cyanosis are directly related to the severity of pulmonary stenosis and the degree of reduction of pulmonary blood flow.

131

Patients with tetralogy of Fallot describe three characteristic symptom complexes. First, the degree of cyanosis and the symptoms are variable; any event that lowers systemic vascular resistance increases the right-to-left shunt and leads to symptoms associated with hypoxemia. Exercise, meals, and hot weather, for example, lower systemic vascular resistance, increase right-to-left shunt, and lead to increased cyanosis.

Tetrad spells are another common symptom complex. They consist of episodes in which the child suddenly becomes quite dyspneic and intensely cyanotic. Death due to hypoxia may result unless the spell is properly treated. The mechanism for production of tetrad spells is unknown, but some authors believe they result from contraction of the right ventricular infundibulum, increasing the degree of pulmonary stenosis. This theory is supported by observations that β-adrenergic blocking agents, such as propranolol, by decreasing myocardial contractility, relieve the symptoms. Other evidence suggests that a fall in systemic vascular resistance could also play a role in the production of the spells, and others attribute them to hyperpnea, per se.

Squatting is the third common symptom complex and is virtually diagnostic of tetralogy of Fallot. During exercise or exertion, the child will squat to rest. Squatting increases systemic vascular resistance and thereby reduces right-to-left shunt. It also briefly increases the systemic venous return; therefore, right ventricular stroke volume and pulmonary blood flow are improved.

Congestive cardiac failure does not occur in patients with tetralogy of Fallot. The left ventricle handles a normal volume of blood. Although the right ventricle is developing a systemic level of pressure, it tolerates the elevated systolic pressure well, since it has been developing this level of pressure since birth. Furthermore, no matter how severe the pulmonary stenosis, the right ventricular systolic pressure cannot rise above systemic levels because the right ventricle freely communicates with the left ventricle through the ventricular septal defect. Only when another abnormality such as anemia or bacterial endocarditis develops can congestive cardiac failure occur.

Children with tetralogy of Fallot show easy fatigability, and as in all instances of cyanotic heart disease, they may have complications of cerebral thrombosis or brain abscess.

Physical Examination

Physical examination reveals cyanosis and, in older children, clubbing. Cardiac size is normal. The most important auscultatory finding is a harsh ejection murmur located along the mid and upper left sternal border. Depending upon the loudness of the murmur, a thrill may be present. The murmur is caused by the pulmonary stenosis and not by the ventricular septal defect. Although the murmur is not diagnostic of tetralogy of Fallot, the loudness of the murmur is inversely related to the severity of the stenosis. The murmur is softer in patients who have more severe stenosis because the volume of flow through the stenotic area is reduced. This useful clinical fact allows assessment of the severity of the condition and verifies that the murmur originates from the right ventricular outflow area and not from the ventricular septal defect. In patients with coexistent pulmonary valvular atresia, an ejection murmur is not heard, but rather a continuous murmur representing either patent ductus arteriosus or bronchial collateral arteries may be heard over the lung fields.

Electrocardiographic Features

The electrocardiogram reveals right axis deviation, and in more severe cases, right atrial enlargement (Fig. 40). Right ventricular hypertrophy is always present and usually is associated with positive T waves in lead V_1.

Roentgenographic Features

The heart size is normal (Fig. 41). The cardiac contour is characteristic. The heart is boot-shaped ("coeur en sabot"). The apex is turned upward and the pulmonary artery segment is concave because the pulmonary artery is small. On the oblique and lateral views, right ventricular hypertrophy and right atrial enlargement are evident. The aorta is frequently enlarged, and in at least 25 percent of the cases a right aortic arch is present.

Summary of Clinical Findings

The history and roentgenographic findings are usually quite diagnostic of tetralogy of Fallot. Once this diagnosis has been made, the loudness of the

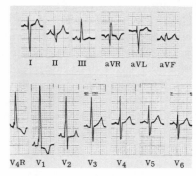

Figure 40. Electrocardiogram in tetralogy of Fallot. QRS axis of 150°. Right ventricular hypertrophy indicated by tall R wave in leads V_4R and V_1 and deep S wave in lead V_6.

133

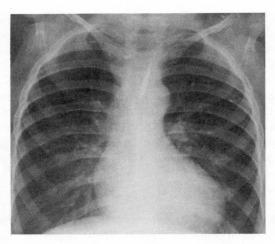

Figure 41. Thoracic roentgenogram in tetralogy of Fallot. Normal-sized heart and decreased pulmonary vasculature. Prominent aortic knob, concave pulmonary artery segment.

murmur, character, severity and frequency of symptoms, and level of hemoglobin and hematocrit provide the most reliable indications of the patient's course.

Natural History

Symptoms progress in patients with tetralogy of Fallot because of increasing infundibular stenosis. Increasing frequency or severity of symptoms, rising hemoglobin, and decreasing intensity of the murmur are signs of progression. The electrocardiogram and roentgenogram show no change, however.

Cardiac Catheterization

The oxygen values through the right side of the heart show no evidence of a left-to-right shunt. Desaturation of aortic blood is found. A pressure drop is found across the outflow area of the right ventricle; the body of the right ventricle has the same pressure as the left ventricle and the pulmonary arterial pressure is lower than normal.

Right ventricular angiography is needed to define the anatomic details of the right ventricular outflow area. Such studies demonstrate the site of the stenosis in the right ventricle, define the pulmonary arterial tree, and show opacification of the aorta through the ventricular septal defect.

Medical Management

As in all patients with cyanotic forms of congenital heart disease, the development of iron deficiency anemia must be prevented or promptly treated when it develops because increased symptoms can occur in anemic patients. Infants and children with tetrad spells should be treated by the administration of 100 percent oxygen and by placing the child in a knee-chest position. Morphine or propranolol is also indicated.

Operative Considerations

A variety of operations are available for children with tetralogy of Fallot. Three types of palliative procedures are available: Blalock-Taussig shunt (anastomosing a subclavian artery to the pulmonary arteries), Waterston shunt (creating a communication between the right pulmonary artery and the ascending aorta), or Potts procedure (creating a communication between the left pulmonary artery and the descending aorta). These are indicated in infants with significant symptoms such as marked cyanosis or hypoxia. These procedures are also indicated in older children with tetralogy of Fallot in whom the pulmonary arteries are too small for corrective operation. Each of these operations allows an increased volume of pulmonary blood flow and an improvement of arterial saturation.

Tetralogy of Fallot can also be corrected by closing the ventricular septal defect and by resecting the pulmonary stenosis. Corrective operations are usually performed in preschool children. There is now a tendency to perform corrective procedures in symptomatic infants, rather than performing a palliative procedure. In older children the operative mortality is around 5 percent, but it is higher in infants. Postoperatively, many patients need to be treated for congestive cardiac failure developing as a consequence of the right ventriculotomy and because of residual cardiac anomalies such as persistent outflow obstruction or ventricular septal defect. Despite the corrective operations for tetralogy of Fallot that have been performed for a number of years, the results are still not entirely satisfactory. Some patients may require reoperation for residual anomalies.

Summary

Tetralogy of Fallot accounts for 75 percent of the cases of cyanotic heart disease in children over the age of 2 years. The symptoms and roentgenographic features are characteristic. Several signs and symptoms permit the evaluation of the natural progression of pulmonary stenosis. Several types of operations are available, but restoration to a truly normal state is the exception.

TRICUSPID ATRESIA

In this malformation (Fig. 42), the tricuspid valve and the inflow portion of the right ventricle do not develop, so that no direct communication exists

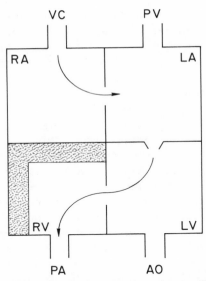

Figure 42. Central circulation in tricuspid atresia and normally related great vessels.

between the right atrium and the right ventricle. Therefore, the circulation is severely altered. The systemic venous return entering the right atrium flows entirely in a right-to-left direction into the left atrium through either an atrial septal defect or a patent foramen ovale.

In the left atrium the systemic venous return mixes with the pulmonary venous blood and is delivered to the left ventricle. The left ventricle ejects blood into the aorta and through a ventricular septal defect into a rudimentary right ventricle and then into the pulmonary artery. Usually the ventricular septal defect is small. The right ventricle is hypoplastic and frequently pulmonary stenosis coexists. Therefore, a high degree of resistance to blood flow into the lungs is present. In most patients with tricuspid atresia, the pulmonary blood flow is reduced.

In one quarter of patients with tricuspid atresia, transposition of the great vessels coexists; therefore, the pulmonary artery arises from the left ventricle and the aorta arises from the hypoplastic right ventricle. In such patients, the pulmonary blood flow is greatly increased because of the relatively low pulmonary vascular resistance and the increased resistance to systemic blood flow because of the systemic vascular resistance from a small ventricular septal defect and hypoplastic right ventricle.

Rarely, the ventricular septum is intact and the pulmonary valve is atretic, so that pulmonary blood flow is through either a patent ductus arteriosus or the bronchial collateral arteries.

In all forms of tricuspid atresia, both the systemic and pulmonary venous returns mix in the left ventricle; in this sense, tricuspid atresia is also an admixture lesion. Because of this fact, the degree of cyanosis is inversely related to the volume of pulmonary blood flow. Therefore, the patient with tricuspid atresia and normally related great vessels is more cyanotic than the patient with tricuspid atresia and transposition of the great vessels. The degree of cyanosis can be useful in following the course of the patient.

Two aspects of the circulation are important in influencing the course of patients and in directing the therapy. The first concerns the atrial septum. In many patients an atrial septal defect is present; in patients with only a patent foramen ovale (no defect) severe obstruction exists.

The second aspect relates to the volume of pulmonary blood flow. Usually pulmonary blood flow is reduced and the resultant hypoxia and related symptoms require palliation. But patients with markedly increased pulmonary blood flow, almost always related to coexistent transposition of the great vessels, can develop congestive cardiac failure because of volume overload of the left ventricle.

History

Children with tricuspid atresia are generally symptomatic in infancy and show cyanosis. Hypoxic spells may be present but squatting is rare. In the patient with increased pulmonary blood flow, cyanosis may be slight, and the dominant clinical features relate to congestive cardiac failure. An unusual patient with the "proper" amount of pulmonary stenosis may be relatively asymptomatic for years.

Physical Examination

The physical findings are not diagnostic of tricuspid atresia. Cyanosis is generally evident and frequently intense. The liver may be enlarged if there is congestive cardiac failure or an obstructing atrial communication. In a third of the cases, either no murmur or a very soft murmur is present, indicating marked reduction in pulmonary blood flow. In patients with large ventricular septal defect or with coexistent transposition of the great vessels, a grade III-IV/VI murmur is present along the left sternal border, and in these patients an apical diastolic murmur may also be found. The second heart sound is single.

Electrocardiographic Features

The electrocardiographic findings are usually diagnostic of tricuspid atresia (Fig. 43). Left axis deviation is almost uniformly present and is usually between 0° and −60°. Tall, peaked P waves of right atrial enlargement and a short PR interval are common features. Because the right

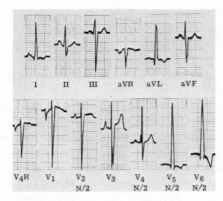

Figure 43. Electrocardiogram in tricuspid atresia. Left axis deviation of QRS complex ($-30°$). P waves broad and notched in lead I indicate left atrial enlargement. Pattern of left ventricular hypertrophy with deep S wave in lead V_1 and tall R wave in lead V_6. N/2 = half-standardization.

ventricle is rudimentary, it contributes little to the total electrical forces forming the QRS complex. The precordial leads show a pattern of left ventricular hypertrophy with an rS complex in lead V_1 and a tall R wave in V_6. This precordial pattern is particularly striking in infancy because of the marked difference from the normal infantile pattern of tall R waves in the right precordium. In older patients the T waves become inverted in the left precordial leads.

Roentgenographic Features

The pulmonary vasculature is decreased in most patients, but it is, of course, increased in those with coexistent transposition of the great vessels or large ventricular septal defect. Cardiac size is almost always increased because of the increased right atrial size and the prominent left ventricle. The cardiac contour is highly suggestive of tricuspid atresia because of the prominent right heart border (enlarged right atrium) and the prominent left heart border (prominent left ventricle).

Summary of Clinical Findings

In patients with cyanosis, the electrocardiogram presents the most important diagnostic clue. The combination of left axis deviation and pattern of left ventricular hypertrophy is highly suggestive of tricuspid atresia. The roentgenographic findings are also helpful if the pulmonary vasculature is decreased.

The auscultatory findings and history are not diagnostic but do provide clues for the severity of the conditions.

Cardiac Catheterization

Oximetry data reveal a right-to-left shunt at the atrial level. The oxygen values in the left ventricle, aorta, and pulmonary artery are similar and are inversely related to pulmonary blood flow. In some cases the right atrial pressure is elevated, indicating a restricted interatrial communication.

Definitive diagnosis depends upon angiographic demonstration of a right-to-left shunt at the atrial level and failure to demonstrate the right ventricle on the early films. Left ventriculography shows simultaneous opacification of both great vessels and permits the identification of obstruction to pulmonary blood flow.

At the time of cardiac catheterization, if done in infancy, a balloon atrial septostomy is frequently performed to reduce obstruction to flow into the left atrium.

Operative Considerations

Various palliative procedures are available for patients with tricuspid atresia. In infants with reduced pulmonary blood flow, a Waterston shunt (right pulmonary artery-ascending aorta) is performed, often combined with a Blalock-Hanlon (atrial septostomy) shunt. Blalock-Taussig shunts are performed in older children. Some centers prefer a Glenn procedure (anastomosis is between the superior vena cava and the pulmonary artery) after 1 year of age.

In children with increased pulmonary blood flow, pulmonary arterial banding is indicated.

Another operation (Fontan procedure) is available for older patients with tricuspid atresia and normally related great vessels. A valved conduit is inserted between the right atrium and the pulmonary artery, and the atrial defect is closed. The long-term results of the procedure are yet to be evaluated.

Summary

Children with tricuspid atresia present with cyanosis and cardiac failure. A murmur may or may not be present. The electrocardiogram reveals left axis deviation, right atrial enlargement, and left ventricular hypertrophy. Roentgenograms show right atrial and left ventricular enlargement. Palliative and corrective operations are available.

PULMONARY ATRESIA

In this malformation (Fig 44), the pulmonary valve is atretic and the right ventricle is usually hypoplastic. Therefore, there is no direct blood flow

139

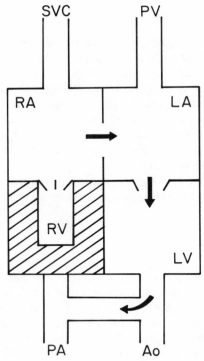

Figure 44. Central circulation in pulmonary atresia.

from the right ventricle to the pulmonary artery. An atrial communication, either foramen ovale or atrial septal defect, is present that allows a right-to-left shunt. Pulmonary blood flow is totally dependent upon patent ductus arteriosus. As the ductus arteriosus closes in the neonatal period, the infant becomes progressively more hypoxic.

History

These patients present in the neonatal period with progressive cyanosis and its complications. Features of congestive cardiac failure are usually not present, although hepatomegaly may be found if the atrial communication is small.

Physical Examination

The infant presents with intense cyanosis and dyspnea. In many patients no murmur is present, but in some a soft continuous murmur of patent ductus arteriosus is found. The second heart sound is single.

Electrocardiographic Features

The electrocardiogram usually shows a normal QRS axis. Peaked P waves of right atrial enlargement are usually present. Since the right ventricle is hypoplastic, the precordial leads show an rS complex in lead V_1 and an R wave in lead V_6. This pattern resembles left ventricular hypertrophy and is in striking contrast to the normal pattern for a newborn. The T waves are usually normal.

Roentgenographic Features

The pulmonary vasculature is reduced. The cardiac contour resembles tricuspid atresia in showing prominent right atrial and left ventricular borders. The cardiac size is always enlarged.

Summary of Clinical Findings

In a cyanotic infant, the combination of roentgenographic findings of cardiomegaly and reduced pulmonary vascular markings and left ventricular hypertrophy on electrocardiogram suggests the diagnosis of pulmonary atresia. It may be distinguished from tricuspid atresia by the difference in the QRS axis, but this is not completely reliable.

Cardiac Catheterization

The oxygen saturation shows a right-to-left shunt at the atrial level and often marked systemic arterial oxygen desaturation because of severe limitation of pulmonary blood flow. The right atrial pressure is often elevated because of a narrowed atrial communication. The hypoplastic right ventricle can be entered; a high pressure may be recorded.

Right atrial angiography shows a right-to-left shunt at the atrial level and resembles tricuspid atresia. Left ventriculography usually distinguishes these conditions because the ventricular septal defect and right ventricular outflow areas are not seen in pulmonary atresia, but rather the aorta is opacified and subsequently the pulmonary artery is visualized by a patent ductus arteriosus. The right ventricle may be injected very cautiously, by hand, and with small volume. This may allow the determination of the distance between the right ventricle cavity and the main pulmonary artery (filled from the ductus on separate injection).

Operative Considerations

These patients require an emergency operation in the neonatal period. Usually a Waterston procedure is performed, combined with a Blalock-

Hanlon procedure. The risk is high because many of the infants are in critical condition at the time of operation. In survivors, a pulmonary valvotomy can be performed subsequently, in the hope that the hypoplastic right ventricle will increase in size.

Summary

Pulmonary atresia resembles tricuspid atresia with normally related great vessels in hemodynamics, clinical and laboratory findings, and operative considerations. In both conditions the severity of symptoms is related to the adequacy of the communication between the atria and the volume of pulmonary blood flow. The conditions can be distinguished by the difference in the QRS axis.

EBSTEIN'S MALFORMATION OF THE TRICUSPID VALVE

In Ebstein's malformation (Fig. 45), the leaflets of the tricuspid valve attach to the right ventricular wall rather than to the tricuspid valve annulus. The tricuspid valve is displaced into the right ventricle, so a portion of the right ventricle between the tricuspid annulus and the displaced tricuspid valve forms part of the right atrial chamber. An atrial septal defect is usually a component of the malformation.

The malformation has two hemodynamic consequences. First, the tricuspid valve frequently permits tricuspid regurgitation. Secondly, the

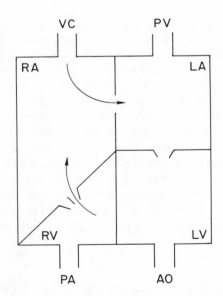

Figure 45. Central circulation in Ebstein's malformation of the tricuspid valve.

portion of the right ventricle between the tricuspid and pulmonary valves is small and noncompliant. As a result, right ventricular inflow is impeded so a right-to-left shunt exists at the atrial level and pulmonary blood flow is decreased.

History

Patients frequently have a history of cyanosis in the first week of life (as in atrial septal defect) and then may appear acyanotic or minimally cyanotic for a variable period, only to become cyanotic later in life. As pulmonary vascular resistance decreases in the neonatal period, the symptomatic newborn may improve due to a decrease in resistance to pulmonary blood flow. Cyanosis is greater in patients whose valve is more deformed and farther displaced into the right ventricle. Congestive cardiac failure may also be present in those with more severe forms and, transiently, in neonates with a less abnormal anatomy. Episodes of rapid heart action, either paroxysmal atrial tachycardia or atrial flutter, may occur and are related to the right atrial dilatation, and in some, to preexcitation (Wolff-Parkinson-White syndrome).

Physical Examination

Cyanosis may be minimal or absent. There may be a precordial bulge. The auscultatory findings are characteristic. A quadruple rhythm is often present. Both the first and second heart sounds are split. A fourth heart sound may be present. There is usually a systolic murmur of variable intensity, indicating tricuspid insufficiency. In addition, a rough diastolic murmur is often heard in the tricuspid area.

Electrocardiographic Features

The electrocardiographic features are characteristic of this condition (Fig. 46). Right atrial enlargement is evident and the P wave may be 8 or 9 mm in height. The QRS duration is prolonged because of complete right bundle branch block. Wolff-Parkinson-White syndrome is present in 20 percent of patients. The precordial leads show a pattern of ventricular hypertrophy, and the R wave in lead V_1 rarely exceeds 10 mm in height.

Roentgenographic Features

The heart is enlarged and may have a boxlike configuration. The right atrium is enlarged. The pulmonary vascular markings are diminished.

143

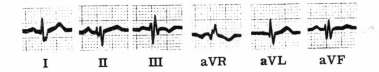

I II III aVR aVL aVF

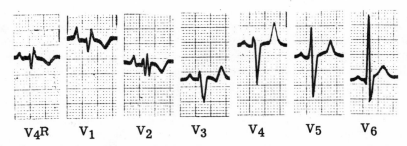

V₄R V₁ V₂ V₃ V₄ V₅ V₆

Figure 46. Electrocardiogram in Ebstein's malformation of the tricuspid valve. Indeterminate QRS axis in the frontal plane. Peaked P waves in lead V_1 indicate right atrial enlargement. QRS complexes in precordial leads show complete right bundle branch block with a broad rSR' pattern evident in leads V_4R and V_1.

Cardiac Catheterization

The oximetry data show a right-to-left shunt at the atrial level. Right ventricular pressure is normal, while right atrial pressure is elevated. Angiography may be diagnostic in showing the abnormal position of the tricuspid valve, the enlarged right atrium, and the right-to-left atrial shunt. Arrhythmias are common during catheterization and must be monitored carefully and treated promptly.

Operative Considerations

The preferred operation is a shunt procedure for those patients with markedly reduced pulmonary blood flow, although in a few patients a prosthetic valve can be placed in the tricuspid annulus, particularly for those with congestive failure.

Summary

The diagnosis of Ebstein's malformation can usually be made clinically because of the history and auscultatory and electrocardiographic findings. Palliative procedures are available.

144

OTHER CONGENITAL CARDIAC ANOMALIES

Congenitally Corrected Transposition of the Great Arteries

As said earlier, the term transposition means a reversal of anteroposterior anatomic relationships. Therefore, in transposition of the great arteries, the aorta arises anteriorly and the pulmonary artery arises posteriorly; normally, the anterior blood vessels arise from the infundibulum, which is the outflow portion of the morphologic right ventricle.

In congenitally corrected transposition of the great arteries, these anatomic relationships are present, but the circulation is physiologically correct, i.e., systemic venous return is delivered to the pulmonary arteries and pulmonary venous return is delivered to the aorta.

The anatomy of congenitally corrected transposition of the great arteries differs from complete transposition of the great arteries because inversion of the ventricles coexists. The term *inversion* indicates an anatomic change in the left-right relationships. Therefore, inversion of the ventricles indicates that the morphologic right ventricle lies on the left side and the morphologic left ventricle lies on the right side. It is the inversion of the ventricles in corrected transposition of the great arteries that allows the circulation to flow in a normal pattern.

In Figure 47, the anatomy of corrected transposition of the great arteries is shown. The systemic venous return from the inferior and superior venae cavae passes into the normally positioned right atrium. This blood then flows into a ventricle that has the following morphologic features of a left ventricle. It has a mitral valve, is a smooth-walled chamber, and there is fibrous continuity between the atrioventricular and semilunar valves, which in this instance are mitral and pulmonary. This ventricle is located to the right of the other ventricle. This anatomic left ventricle ejects blood into a posteriorly and medially placed pulmonary trunk (as anticipated in transposition).

The pulmonary venous blood returns into the normally placed left atrium. The flow then crosses the tricuspid valve into a ventricle having the morphologic features of a right ventricle. It is trabeculated, has a tricuspid valve, and the atrioventricular and semilunar valves are separated by an infundibulum. The aorta arises from the infundibulum and lies anteriorly and laterally to the pulmonary trunk.

The circulation, therefore, in this cardiac anomaly is normal, and the anatomic relationship of the great vessels fulfills the definition of transposition of the great arteries. This type of transposition has also been termed l-transposition because the aorta lies to the left of the pulmonary artery.

145

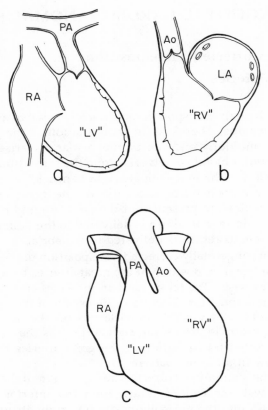

Figure 47. Congenitally corrected transposition of the great vessels. A. Diagram of anatomic relationships of the right side of the heart. Right atrium (RA) communicates with anatomic left ventricle ("LV") through mitral valve. This ventricle connects with the pulmonary artery (PA). Note continuity between mitral and pulmonary valves. B. Diagram of anatomic relationships of left side of heart. Left atrium (LA) communicates through tricuspid valve with anatomic right ventricle ("RV"). This connects with aorta (Ao). Note tricuspid and aortic valves separated by an infundibulum. C. External configuration of heart and great vessels.

This condition would lead to no cardiovascular symptoms or murmurs, but in virtually all patients other cardiac anomalies coexist. Ventricular septal defect, pulmonary stenosis, and insufficiency of the left-sided atrioventricular valve are the most common cardiac anomalies in these patients.

These coexistent anomalies lead to clinical and laboratory findings similar to those found in patients with the same anomaly but with normal relationships between the ventricles and the great vessels. Three clinical findings, however, allow detection of congenitally corrected transposition of the great arteries as the underlying cardiac malformation.

1. The second heart sound along the upper left sternal border is loud and single. Because the aorta is located anteriorly and leftward, the aortic valve lies immediately beneath this area. The second sound appears single because the pulmonary valve is distant (posteriorly positioned), so its component is inaudible.

2. On thoracic roentgenogram, the left cardiac border is straight or shows only two rounded contours, in contrast to that in patients with normally related great vessels, in which three contours—aortic knob, pulmonary trunk, and left ventricular border—are present.

3. The third distinctive clinical feature relates to ventricular inversion. The bundles of His are also inverted, so the ventricular septum depolarizes from right to left, the opposite direction of normal. This leads to a q wave in lead V_1 and an initial positive deflection in lead V_6. The precordial lead pattern is opposite the normal pattern of an initial r wave in lead V_1 and a q wave in lead V_6. Such a pattern is present in almost all patients with congenitally corrected transposition of the great arteries. A word of caution: patients with severe right ventricular hypertrophy may also show such a pattern, so this electrocardiographic finding alone does not diagnose corrected transposition of the great arteries. Patients with congenitally corrected transposition of the great arteries tend to spontaneously develop partial or complete heart block.

Our understanding of the development of congenitally corrected transposition of the great arteries is incomplete, but the anomaly is believed to result from looping of the cardiac tube to the left rather than, as is normal, to the right (Fig. 48). Thus the "right ventricle" is positioned to the left and the left ventricle is located medially, leading to the ventricular inversion. Apparently this malrotation of the cardiac tube also leads to the abnormal position of the great arteries.

Malposition of the Heart

The heart may assume an abnormal position in the thorax and be in either the left or the right side of the chest. Various classifications of cardiac malposition have been developed, but we favor the one presented here, although the terminology may be different from that of other authors.

Certain anatomic features are important in understanding cardiac malpositions. In normal patients and virtually all those with cardiac malposition, certain anatomic relations are constant: 1) the inferior vena cava (at the diaphragm), the anatomic right atrium, and the major lobe of the liver are located on one side of the body; while 2) the aorta (at the diaphragm), the anatomic left atrium, and the stomach are located on the opposite side of the body. Consider the anatomic relationships in the normal individual wherein the liver, inferior vena cava, and right atrium are present on the right side of the body; while the stomach, aorta, and left atrium are pres-

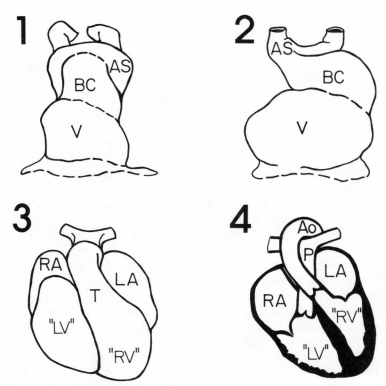

Figure 48. Diagram of developmental aspects of inversion of the ventricles in congenitally corrected transposition of the great vessels. Primitive bulboventricular loop rotates toward left (1 and 2) instead of normal direction toward the right. This leads to the inversion of the ventricles. The anatomic left ventricle relating to the right atrium and the anatomic right ventricle relating to the left atrium. AS = aortic sinus. BC = bulbocordis. V = ventricularis. RA = right atrium. LA = left atrium. "RV" = anatomic right ventricle. "LV" = anatomic left ventricle. T = truncus arteriosus. Ao = aorta. P = pulmonary artery.

ent on the left side. This relationship is called *situs solitus* (Fig. 49). The inferior vena cava is crucial in our considerations as it is an important link between the abdominal and thoracic contents.

DEXTROCARDIA

Dextrocardia is a general term indicating that the cardiac apex is located in the right side of the chest. Three anatomic variations associated with dextrocardia are presented here.

Situs Inversus Heart

This condition is the opposite of the usual situs solitus (Fig. 49). The inferior vena cava, the major lobe of the liver, and the right atrium are

Dextrocardia

Levocardia

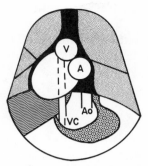

Dextroposition
(Situs Solitus)

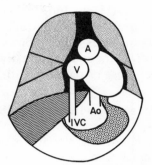

Levoposition
(Situs Solitus)

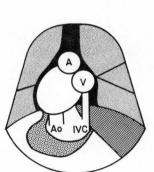

Situs Inversus

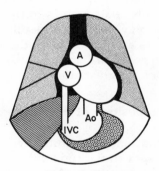

Situs Solitus

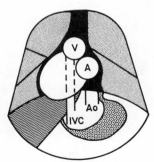

Dextroversion
(Situs Solitus)

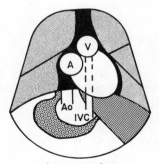

Levoversion
(Situs Inversus)

Figure 49. Diagrams of malposition of the heart. Ao = aorta. IVC = inferior vena cava. V = venous atrium. A = arterial atrium.

located on the left side of the body. This has also been termed mirror-image dextrocardia, because the anatomic relationships are exactly the reverse of normal. Other anatomic findings include the presence of two lobes in the right lung, three lobes in the left lung, and the appendix located in the left lower quadrant.

Situs inversus heart is probably associated with an increased incidence of cardiac anomalies, but the type and distribution of the anomalies parallel those of patients with situs solitus.

Dextroversion with Situs Solitus

In this condition, the anatomic relationships of situs solitus are present, but the cardiac apex is directed toward the right (Fig. 49). The atria are anchored by the venae cavae, but the ventricles can rotate on the long axis of the heart and lie in the midline or right chest. In dextroversion, the heart may show one of two anatomic forms. In the first, the ventricles are normally related, and ventricular septal defect and pulmonary stenosis are commonly found. In the other form, corrected transposition of the great arteries and inversion of the ventricles are present. These patients show the type of cardiac anomalies commonly found with corrected transposition of the great arteries.

Dextroposition of the Heart

This is another condition with the situs solitus relationship and the cardiac apex in the right side of the chest (Fig. 49). In this instance, cardiac displacement toward the right is caused by extrinsic factors such as hypoplasia of the right lung. In most patients with dextroposition of the heart, cardiac anomalies coexist. The anomalies are often associated with a left-to-right shunt; the patients develop pulmonary vascular disease.

LEVOCARDIA

Levocardia is a general term indicating that the cardiac apex is located in the left side of the chest. Situs solitus is one form of levocardia, but the cardiac apex may also be located abnormally in the left side of the chest.

Levoversion of Situs Inversus

This anatomic relationship is the opposite of dextroversion of situs solitus (Fig. 49). The basic anatomic relationship is situs inversus, but the cardiac apex is located in the left side of the chest. As might be expected, many of these patients have corrected transposition of the great arteries.

150

Levoposition

In patients with situs solitus, the left lung may be hypoplastic, so the heart is displaced farther into the left hemithorax than normal. When this condition exists in a patient with a cardiac anomaly, there is a tendency to develop pulmonary vascular disease.

In each of the conditions discussed above, normal anatomic relationships are present among the inferior vena cava, liver, and right atrium, and among the descending aorta, stomach, and left atrium. There are unusual conditions associated with cardiac malposition in which these anatomic relationships are not present and in which the spleen is abnormal. These conditions have been named after the type of splenic anomaly.

ASPLENIA SYNDROME

In this syndrome the heart may be located in either the left or the right side of the chest, and the spleen is absent. In these patients there are numerous visceral and cardiac anomalies. The visceral anomalies reflect a tendency toward symmetrical organ development, with paired organs each having the form of the right-sided organ, and left-sided structures being absent. Thus, each lung has three lobes (like a right lung), the spleen, a left-sided structure, is absent, and the liver is symmetrical. There is often malrotation of the bowel.

Cardiac anomalies are complex and include atrial and ventricular septal defects, often in the form of endocardial cushion defect; severe pulmonary stenosis or atresia; transposition of the great arteries; and often total anomalous pulmonary venous connection. This combination of anomalies leads to clinical and roentgenographic features that resemble severe tetralogy of Fallot. Despite a palliative procedure, the outlook for these patients is bleak.

Because of the symmetry of the liver, malrotation of the bowel, and midline position of the inferior vena cava, the important anatomic relationships that allow definition of situs are disrupted, so it is difficult to classify the type of cardiac malposition in patients with asplenia.

Polysplenia Syndrome

In this syndrome, as in asplenia, the heart may be located in either the left or the right side of the chest. The spleen is present but is divided into multiple masses. There is also a tendency to symmetrical organ development, in this case bilateral left-sidedness—both lungs appearing as the left lung—and the gallbladder is absent. There is often malrotation of the bowel.

Cardiac anomalies include atrial and/or ventricular septal defect, partial anomalous pulmonary venous connection, and interrupted inferior vena

151

cava with azygous continuation.

The clinical picture resembles that of left-to-right shunt. The prognosis is good and many patients undergo corrective operation.

As in asplenia, difficulty is encountered in determining situs because of the malrotation of the bowel and the fact that the inferior vena cava is interrupted at the level of the diaphragm.

Vascular Ring

Normally, no vascular structure passes behind the esophagus, but there are anomalies wherein the aortic arch or a major arch vessel lies behind the esophagus; this is called vascular ring.

An understanding of the anatomic variations of vascular ring can be gained by studying the development of the aortic arch (Fig. 50). Early in embryonic development the ascending aorta gives rise to a right and a left aortic arch. These arches encircle the trachea and the esophagus and join to form the descending aorta. In addition, there is both a left and a right ductus arteriosus.

In the normal development, the right arch is interrupted beyond the right subclavian artery and the right ductus arteriosus regresses. This leads to a left aortic arch. The proximal portion of the primitive right arch becomes the innominate artery, which in turn gives rise to the right carotid and right subclavian arteries. The other aortic arch vessels are the left carotid and left subclavian arteries. The left ductus arteriosus persists, connecting the aortic arch opposite the left subclavian to the left pulmonary artery.

If the left aortic arch is interrupted beyond the left subclavian artery, the opposite is formed, a right aortic arch with mirror-image branching (Fig. 50). The ascending aorta arises; the first branch is an innominate artery representing the proximal portion of the left aortic arch. From this arise the left subclavian and left carotid arteries. The aortic arch passes toward the right and gives rise to the right carotid and right subclavian arteries. The ductus arteriosus may be on either the left or the right side.

Rarely, neither aortic arch is interrupted during embryonic life. The resultant anomaly is one form of vascular ring—double aortic arch. The ascending aorta divides into two aortic arches. One of the aortic arches passes anteriorly to the trachea and the other passes posteriorly to the esophagus. They join to form the descending aorta that may then pass on either the left or the right side of the thorax. The trachea and esophagus are encircled by vascular structures and can be compressed, leading to respiratory symptoms and difficulty in swallowing.

Two other types of vascular ring can be formed by faulty interruption of one of the aortic arches. If the right aortic arch is interrupted between the right carotid and right subclavian arteries, the aortic arch is left-sided,

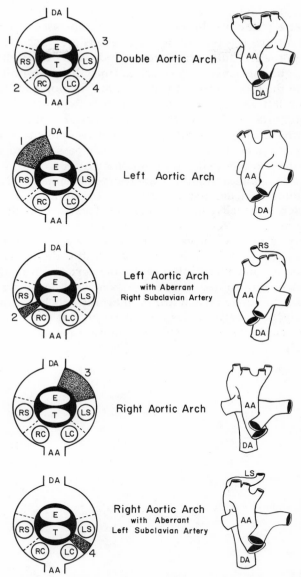

Figure 50. Diagram of development of aortic arch anomalies based on concept of primitive double aortic arch and the resultant aortic arch pattern. The primitive double aortic arch may be uninterrupted developmentally and a double arch results. It may also be interrupted at any of four locations (1-4). These result respectively in a normal left aortic arch, and left aortic arch with aberrant right subclavian artery; right aortic arch, and right aortic arch with aberrant left subclavian artery. AA = ascending aorta. DA = descending aorta. LC = left carotid artery. LS = left subclavian artery. RC = right carotid artery. RS = right subclavian artery. E = esophagus. T = trachea.

but the right subclavian artery is aberrant. In this anomaly, there is no innominate artery; the first branch arising from the ascending aorta is the right carotid artery. The remaining arch vessels are, respectively: the left carotid artery, the left subclavian artery, and finally the right subclavian artery. The right subclavian artery arises from the descending aorta and passes behind the esophagus to the right arm. The opposite situation may develop if the left aortic arch is interrupted between the left subclavian and left carotid arteries. This forms a right aortic arch and an aberrant left subclavian artery. The vascular ring is often completed by a ductus arteriosus, either ligamentous or patent, which passes from the aberrant subclavian artery to the ipsilateral pulmonary artery.

Thus, vascular rings formed by aberrant subclavian arteries can also cause symptoms that are usually relieved by dividing the ductus arteriosus, which is usually ligamentous. Most patients with this form of vascular ring are, however, asymptomatic and require no treatment.

In summary, a number of variations in aortic arch anatomy exist, depending upon the site(s) of interruption of the developmental aortic arches. If they are not interrupted, a double aortic arch is formed. If the aortic arches are interrupted at one site, a normal aortic arch or a right aortic arch, or an aortic arch with an aberrant subclavian artery can be formed. Rarely, the aortic arches are interrupted at two sites, yielding a number of anatomic variations. This last condition is called interruption of the aortic arch.

4

ACQUIRED CARDIAC CONDITIONS

ACUTE RHEUMATIC FEVER

Rheumatic fever is a systemic disease, affecting several organ systems, including the heart. It is a sequel of group A β-hemolytic streptococcal infections, usually tonsillopharyngitis. In less than 1 percent of patients with streptococcal infection, rheumatic fever develops, but the pathogenesis is unknown. Rheumatic fever usually develops 10 days to 2 weeks following a streptococcal pharyngitis that almost always is associated with fever greater than 101°F, sore throat, and cervical adenitis.

Rheumatic fever is diagnosed by application of the modified Jones criteria. These criteria comprise the various combinations of clinical and laboratory manifestations reflecting the multiple sites of disease involvement; there must be two major criteria or one major and two minor criteria, plus evidence of a preceding streptococcal infection, in order to diagnose acute rheumatic fever.

The proof of streptococcal infection can be established by either of two methods. The first is the recovery of β-hemolytic streptococcus by throat culture. This must be interpreted with care because streptococcal carrier states do exist and are not considered a streptococcal infection. The second method of proof is the finding of an increase in streptococcal antibody. Following a streptococcal infection, antibodies to various streptococcal components such as antistreptolysin-O titer, DNase B, and DPNase rise significantly. Titers for several antibodies should be measured because an individual may not form antibodies to each streptococcal product. Almost all instances of streptococcal infection can be identified by elevation of one of these three antibodies. Significant antibody rise indicates a preceding streptococcal infection and is more meaningful than isolating β-hemolytic streptococcus on a throat culture.

There are five major and five minor criteria that can be used to fulfill the Jones criteria, and these give an indication of the pathologic involvement in acute rheumatic fever and the clinical and laboratory manifestations of this disease.

Major Criteria

Carditis

Any layer of the heart may be involved during the course of rheumatic fever. Pericarditis can occur in this disease and can be suspected by the occurrence of chest pain that may be referred to the abdomen or shoulders. It is diagnosed by finding a pericardial friction rub or ST segment elevation on the electrocardiogram.

Cardiac enlargement or cardiac failure without evidence of valvular anomalies is evidence of myocardial involvement. Rarely, cardiac failure occurs from myocardial involvement itself. Various degrees of heart block, gallop rhythm, and muffled heart sounds are other manifestations of myocarditis. Prolonged PR interval in itself is not a criterion for carditis.

Valvular or endocardial involvement of the heart is the most serious manifestation of carditis because it can lead to permanent cardiac sequelae. Both the aortic and mitral valves may be involved acutely. Three types of murmurs may be present that suggest acute rheumatic fever. 1. An apical pansystolic murmur of mitral insufficiency is the most frequently occurring murmur. 2. At times a mid-diastolic murmur may also be heard at the apex. The origin of this murmur is unknown but it is related to turbulence either from the valvulitis or from the blood flow into a dilated left ventricle. 3. A murmur of aortic insufficiency may be found during the acute episode but is a more frequent late manifestation. Aortic stenosis does not occur during the acute episode of rheumatic fever.

Arthritis

Arthritis is another major manifestation of acute rheumatic fever. The arthritis is usually a migrating polyarthritis; several joints may be involved, often sequentially, but at a given time there may be involvement of only one joint. Usually the large joints are involved. Diagnosis of arthritis rests on finding warm and tender joints that are painful on movement. The changes are never permanent.

Chorea

Chorea is a late manifestation of rheumatic fever and often develops several months after the streptococcal infection. At that time, other manifestations of rheumatic fever may not be found. The presence of chorea alone is sufficient for the diagnosis of rheumatic fever. This manifestation is more common in females and prior to puberty.

Chorea is characterized by involuntary, nonrepetitive, purposeless motions, often associated with emotional instability. The parents may complain that their child is clumsy, fidgety, cries easily or has difficulty in writing or reading.

There are classic physical findings of chorea. The milkmaid (or grip) sign describes the fibrillatory nature of a hand grasp. Other findings are related to exaggerated muscle movements such as the hyperextension of the hands or apposition of the backs of the hands when the arms are extended above the head. Although lasting for months in some children, it is not a permanent problem.

Erythema Marginatum

This is a fleeting, characteristic cutaneous finding. It is characterized by pink macules with distinct sharp margins; these change rapidly in contour. Warmth tends to bring out these lesions. With time the center fades, while the margin persists as a circular or serpentine border.

Subcutaneous Nodules

This is a rare manifestation of rheumatic fever, occurring late in the disease course. These are nontender, firm, pealike nodules over the extensor surfaces, particularly over the knees, elbows, and spine. They have a strong association with chronic carditis.

Minor Criteria

Arthralgia

The description of pain in joints without subjective evidence of arthritis may be used as a minor criterion, provided arthritis has not been used as a major one.

Prolonged PR Interval

Prolongation of the PR interval can be used as a minor criterion, provided carditis has not been used as a major one.

Acute Phase Reactants

Laboratory evidence of acute inflammation, such as leukocytosis, elevated erythrocyte sedimentation rate, or C-reactive protein, is found in acute rheumatic fever. Any one of these laboratory findings may be used as a minor criterion.

Previous History of Rheumatic Fever

This can be used as a criterion for diagnosis, but care must be taken that the diagnosis of the previous episode of rheumatic fever was carefully made and in itself follows the Jones criteria.

Fever

The temperature is usually in the range of 101° to 102°F.

Treatment

Bed rest should be prescribed for the duration of the acute febrile period of the illness. Then gradual increases in activity should be allowed, provided that there is no recurrence of signs or symptoms. Serial determination of erythrocyte sedimentation rate is helpful in reaching decisions concerning activity levels. The return to full activity may be achieved by 6 weeks in patients with arthritis as the only major criterion, but in those with carditis, 3 months is probably more realistic.

For most patients, salicylates are the preferred medication to reduce the inflammatory response, and they produce a prompt improvement in arthritis. Temperature associated with rheumatic fever returns to normal within a few days. Although salicylates probably do not affect the course of the disease or the carditis, they do provide symptomatic relief. Aspirin is administered in a dose sufficient to achieve a blood salicylate level of 20 to 25 mg/100 ml; usually this dosage is about 20 mg/kg/day. Salicylates are continued until the erythrocyte sedimentation rate is normal, and then the dosage is tapered.

Although cortisone or related agents have been used in the treatment of acute rheumatic fever, there is little convincing evidence that it prevents cardiac valvular damage. It does, however, lead to a more prompt reduction in symptoms than does aspirin. Since steroids are more hazardous, their use should be reserved for patients with severe pancarditis.

The patient with acute rheumatic fever should be treated for β-hemolytic streptococcal infection by the administration of either 1.2 million units of benzathine penicillin or 250,000 units of penicillin G, four times a day for 10 days.

In monitoring the course of the disease, it is not necessary to obtain repeated streptococcal antibody studies, since these values do not parallel the disease course.

Rheumatic Fever Prophylaxis

Once a patient has had an episode of rheumatic fever, he has a higher risk of developing a second episode, particularly in the first 5 years, but some added risk continues throughout life. Since rheumatic fever develops following a streptococcal infection, preventive measures are directed at eliminating such infections in susceptible individuals.

The American Heart Association has recommended that all patients with a history of rheumatic fever be placed on continuous, lifelong penicillin prophylaxis. Penicillin can be administered in two forms: 1) penicillin G, 250,000 units orally twice a day; or 2) benzathine penicillin, 1.2 million units, intramuscularly monthly. If the patient is allergic to penicillin, sulfadiazine, 250 mg twice a day, should be given. Although sulfa drugs are not bactericidal and should not be used for the treatment of a streptococcal infection, they are bacteriostatic for streptococcus and prevent colonization of the nasopharynx.

The current recommendations are for lifelong prophylaxis. After childhood and late adolescent years, the likelihood of patients developing a streptococcal infection is slight; but the cost of prophylaxis is small in relation to the valvular damage that can result from rheumatic fever.

The aim of physicians should be the prevention of the initial episode of rheumatic fever by recognition and proper treatment of group A β-hemolytic streptococcal infections. It is only by adequate treatment of such infections that rheumatic fever can be prevented.

When rheumatic fever occurs, it almost invariably develops as a complication of group A β-hemolytic streptococcal tonsillopharyngitis. Tonsillopharyngitis can result from several etiologic agents other than group A β-hemolytic streptococcus. Streptococcal tonsillopharyngitis is usually associated with fever, cervical adenitis, and exudate on the tonsils, but this is not invariable, and other causes of sore throat such as infectious mononucleosis can show similar findings. Diagnosis of group A β-hemolytic streptococcal tonsillopharyngitis rests on the identification of this organism on throat culture.

The throat of any child with the symptoms and findings of tonsillopharyngitis should be cultured. If β-hemolytic streptococcus is present, the throat culture will be positive within 24 hours. The child with a positive culture should be treated then; it is not necessary to initiate treatment at the time of culturing the child, since antibiotic treatment does not alter the acute course of group A β-hemolytic streptococcal tonsillopharyngitis. The aim of treatment of this infection is the eradication of the streptococcus. This is done by administering penicillin in either of two ways:

1. 1.2 million units of benzathine penicillin or
2. 250,000 units of penicillin G, 4 times a day for 10 days. The intramuscular route is associated with a slightly better rate of eradication and is better for patients in whom compliance may be a factor.

After completion of the course of oral penicillin or 3 weeks after an injection of penicillin, the patient should have a repeat throat culture. If the culture is still positive, retreatment should be undertaken with benzathine penicillin.

In patients allergic to penicillin, erythromycin (0.75 to 1.5 $gm/m_2/24$ hours in 4 divided doses) is the drug of choice.

Long-Term Care

After the acute episode of rheumatic fever, the patient should be seen periodically. The purposes of these visits are to: 1) emphasize the continuing need of penicillin prophylaxis for rheumatic fever; 2) emphasize the need for additional prophylaxis against bacterial endocarditis at the time of dental work or other procedures; and 3) observe for the development of valvular rheumatic heart disease. In half of the patients with evidence of valvular abnormality during the acute episode, the murmurs disappear, but over a period of years the other half may develop more severe cardiac manifestations such as mitral stenosis, mitral insufficiency, or aortic insufficiency. These may require operation.

PRIMARY MYOCARDIAL DISEASES

The term primary myocardial disease encompasses a diffuse group of conditions affecting principally the myocardium and leading to similar clinical and physiologic states. It excludes obvious valvular heart disease, congenital heart disease, hypertension, and coronary arterial disease.

Despite the various etiologic factors of myocardial disease, the major signs and symptoms of primary myocardial diseases are similar. Because of the myocardial involvement, there is failure of the heart to: 1) act as a pump; 2) initiate and maintain its rhythm; and 3) maintain its architecture. Each of these three effects of myocardial involvement has clinical and laboratory findings. The inability of the myocardium to act efficiently as a pump is shown clinically by features of congestion and inadequate forward flow of blood. Prominent are the findings of congestive cardiac failure, pulmonary edema, dyspnea, hepatomegaly, peripheral edema, and gallop rhythm. Symptoms of fatigue, angina, dizziness, and exercise intolerance indicate inadequate systemic output.

Cardiac arrhythmias are common in these patients and indicate another facet of myocardial involvement. Two types of arrhythmias are present. There may be slowing of conduction, particularly through the atrioventricular node, leading to first degree, or more advanced, heart block. Ectopic pacemaker sites may develop, leading to atrial or ventricular tachycardias. Further indications of inadequate electrical activity of the heart include low voltage QRS complexes and abnormalities of the T wave.

Finally, there is the group of signs and symptoms related to the inability of the heart to maintain its normal muscular architecture. The most obvious finding on clinical examination is the displacement of the cardiac apex. Cardiomegaly is also found on the thoracic roentgenogram and may be so extensive as to interfere with the left-sided bronchi. Mitral insufficiency may develop either from dilation of the mitral ring or from papillary muscle dysfunction. Prominent third and fourth heart sounds develop and are related to increased left ventricular filling pressure.

Typically, the patient presents with congestive cardiac failure, cardiomegaly (particularly involving the left side of the heart), and absence of a cardiac murmur.

The primary myocardial diseases are divided into three categories: myocarditis, myocardial disease of obscure origin, and myocardial involvement with systemic disease.

Myocarditis

The myocardium may be involved in an inflammatory process related to infectious agents, collagen disease, or unknown causes. Although many are considered to be of viral origin, this relationship has often been difficult to prove. Echo, Coxsackie, and rubella viruses are identifiable causes of myocarditis in childhood. Myocarditis is generally a disease of the neonatal period or early infancy and occurs sporadically thereafter. In the young age group, the onset may be abrupt, with sudden cardiovascular collapse or the more gradual onset of congestive cardiac failure. The cardiac failure may respond well to treatment. The infant is mottled and has weak peripheral pulses. Evidence of cardiomegaly is found clinically and the heart sounds are muffled. Tachycardia is a regular feature. The electrocardiogram shows normal or reduced QRS voltages. ST segment depression and T wave inversion are positive and are usually found in the left precordial leads. Cardiomegaly and pulmonary congestion are found on the thoracic roentgenogram.

The prognosis is poor in neonates. In older patients, treatment with digitalis usually improves the patient's status, although the course may be chronic with longstanding evidence of cardiomegaly.

Myocardial Disease of Obscure Origin

This diffuse group of diseases of unknown etiology shows no evidence of myocardial inflammation. The major pediatric conditions of this category are: endocardial fibroelastosis, idiopathic myocardial hypertrophy, and familial hypertrophy.

Endocardial Fibroelastosis

Endocardial fibroelastosis is a disease of unknown origin; some believe it results from a viral infection. The endocardium, particularly of the left ventricle and left atrium, is thickened by a proliferation of fibrous and elastic tissue. The endocardium may be 2 mm thick, whereas in the normal individual it is only a few cells thick. The myocardium shows minimal change. The papillary muscles arise high on the left ventricular wall, and this abnormal position contributes to the mitral insufficiency.

The disease usually presents in infancy, with the onset of congestive cardiac failure. The cardiac failure often responds promptly to digitalization. Growth is retarded and there may be frequent respiratory infections. Often a soft systolic murmur is present at the apex, presumably due to the abnormal mitral valve. Electrocardiograms show left ventricular hypertrophy, manifested by tall R waves in the left precordial leads and inverted T waves in these leads. Gross cardiomegaly, particularly of the left atrium and left ventricle, is present on the roentgenogram.

With the use of digitalis preparations, the prognosis for survival during childhood is good, although we have had several children who died in adolescence after a long asymptomatic period. Occasionally the mitral valve needs to be replaced in patients with severe mitral regurgitation.

Idiopathic Hypertrophic Subaortic Stenosis

In this condition the myocardium is greatly thickened; this may involve the ventricles diffusely or only the ventricular septum. During systole the hypertrophied myocardium bulges into the left ventricular outflow tract and may result in subaortic obstruction. Other names for this condition are hypertrophic obstructive cardiomyopathy and asymmetrical septal hypertrophy. If the septum, primarily, is thickened, it may also bulge into the right ventricular outflow tract and cause subpulmonary obstruction as well. The family history may reveal other members with similar conditions.

Syncope and congestive cardiac failure may be present. On physical examination, the peripheral pulses are brisk and palpation of the apex reveals a double impulse. A long systolic murmur is present along the left sternal border and faintly radiates to the base(s). The murmur varies in intensity with change in position. Third and fourth sounds may be present.

Electrocardiograms show a normal QRS axis and occasionally left atrial enlargement and left ventricular hypertrophy, often with ST segment and T wave changes. Deep Q waves may be found in the left precordial leads. Conduction abnormalities of a nonspecific nature may alter the QRS complex.

162

Cardiac enlargement related to the left ventricle and the left atrium is regularly found on the roentgenogram, in contrast to other forms of aortic stenosis. The ascending aorta is normal size.

Because of their inotropic effects, the use of digitalis or isoproterenol, since they increase the gradient, is contraindicated in these patients. Operation involving excision of portions of the septal myocardium has been recommended for some patients, but there are few long-term studies of the procedure.

Myocardial Involvement with Systemic Disease

The myocardium of children with certain generalized diseases may be altered as a result of the particular disease process. Inflammatory changes may occur in conditions such as lupus erythematosus. Abnormal substances may accumulate in the heart, as in glycogen storage disease type II or Hurler's syndrome. Myocardial fibrosis may develop in neuromuscular disease such as Friedreich's ataxia or muscular dystrophy.

Glycogen Storage Disease, Type II

This condition, called Pompe's disease, caused by a deficiency of acid maltase, leads to the accumulation of glycogen in the myocardium, causing it to be thickened to twice normal dimensions.

The infants present with congestive cardiac failure because of the cardiac involvement. Generalized muscular weakness is also prominent clinically because of the skeletal muscle involvement. The liver, which may contain increased glycogen content, may be enlarged out of proportion to the degree of cardiac failure.

Cardiac examination may be unrevealing except for evidence of cardiomegaly. The electrocardiogram is diagnostic and shows greatly increased QRS voltages and often a shortened PR interval. Cardiomegaly, particularly left ventricular enlargement, is found.

The prognosis is poor; death occurs in the first year of life. There is no known form of therapy.

Anomalous Origin of the Left Coronary Artery

In the differential diagnosis of infants with manifestations of primary myocardial disease, i.e., congestive cardiac failure, soft murmur or no murmur, cardiomegaly, and ST and T wave changes on the electrocardiogram, another cardiac condition must also be considered. The anomalous origin of the left coronary artery from the pulmonary trunk leads to similar findings but differs from the others in being a congenital anomaly and one that may be improved by operation.

In this condition, the left coronary artery arises from the pulmonary artery, while the right coronary artery arises normally from the aorta. As a

163

result, the left ventricular myocardium is poorly perfused so that ischemia and infarction occur. Initially the inadequate perfusion is related to the low perfusion pressure of the pulmonary artery. Subsequently, collaterals develop between the high pressure right coronary arterial system and the low pressure left coronary arterial system. In this situation, blood flows from the right coronary arterial system into the left pulmonary artery. The left ventricular myocardium is also poorly perfused because of the run-off of blood into the pulmonary trunk.

The infants are usually asymptomatic in the neonatal period. At age 6 weeks, they typically develop episodes that have been described as angina, wherein the infant cries as in pain, is pale, and perspires profusely. These are of short duration and are believed to represent transient myocardial ischemia. Other children may show no symptoms, but many of the patients have signs and symptoms of congestive cardiac failure.

On physical examination the child usually appears normal. There may be no abnormal auscultatory findings or there may be a soft apical systolic murmur of mitral insufficiency.

The electrocardiogram is usually diagnostic and shows a pattern of anterolateral myocardial infarction, manifested by deep Q waves and inverted T waves in leads I, aVL, V_5, and V_6. In a few cases it may show only left ventricular hypertrophy and strain or a pattern of complete left bundle branch block.

The thoracic roentgenogram reveals cardiomegaly and a left ventricular contour.

Patients with cardiac failure should receive digitalis. There are variable criteria for operation. Whereas it was formerly recommended that the anomalously arising left coronary artery should be ligated in all children with a left-to-right shunt, recently there have been variable recommendations. Some still recommend this procedure for infants whose clinical status is deteriorating, while preferring in other cases to wait until the child is older, when a coronary bypass procedure can be performed.

In infancy, the underlying cause of cardiomyopathy is often indicated by the electrocardiographic findings. Although each of the four most frequent causes of cardiomyopathy is associated with ST segment and T wave changes, the QRS patterns may differ. Myocarditis shows normal or reduced QRS voltages, glycogen storage disease, greatly increased voltages, endocardial fibroelastosis, left ventricular hypertrophy and strain, and anomalous left coronary artery pattern of anterolateral myocardial infarction.

In the older child, there may be other clinical signs and symptoms related to the underlying disease, such as the characteristic facies and habitus of Hurler's syndrome or the presence of the L.E. cell in a patient with myocardial involvement in lupus erythematosus. Often, however, there are no findings that allow an etiologic diagnosis because many cases are of unknown origin.

Therapy of primary myocardial disease is directed at the problems developing from the myocardial involvement. Specific treatment is rarely available for the underlying condition. The major therapeutic efforts are made toward cardiac failure and diminished cardiac output. Digitalis is the keystone of therapy to increase myocardial contractility. Some hesitate to use digitalis preparations in patients with myocardial disease, particularly myocarditis, as there is a belief that these patients are unduly sensitive to digitalis. The usual precautions should be heeded in digitalis administration. Other measures for treatment of congestive cardiac failure, such as diuretics, are indicated as well.

Cardiomyopathies may lead to mitral insufficiency, probably not so much from dilatation of the mitral annulus as from abnormalities of the papillary muscles. Papillary muscle dysfunction may be related to infarction of the muscle or subjacent ventricular wall, or result from ventricular dilatation leading to an abnormal position of the papillary muscle. Regardless of the cause, if major mitral regurgitation results, the left ventricular volume is further increased and congestive cardiac failure may be worsened. In such patients, plication or replacement of the mitral valve may have a strikingly beneficial effect.

Cardiac arrhythmias, either heart block or tachyarrhythmias, may also occur in patients with cardiomyopathy and may require treatment. Heart block may not require treatment if the patient is asymptomatic. Should syncope or congestive cardiac failure worsen, placement of a cardiac pacemaker may be indicated.

Tachyarrhythmias, such as premature ventricular contractions, are usually ventricular in origin; supraventricular tachyarrhythmias, such as atrial flutter or fibrillation, may develop secondary to atrial dilatation. These require treatment if they lead to worsening of the cardiac status.

In many patients with cardiomyopathies, bed rest plays a major role in the treatment. The use of corticosteroids in the therapy of myocarditis remains controversial as there is evidence that they increase viral replication, but they should be considered for use in a deteriorating, near fatal state.

The prognosis of primary myocardial disease as a group is unknown and variable since there are a number of diseases that cause this symptom complex. Without specific etiologic diagnosis, it is difficult to give a precise prognosis. Some conditions such as idiopathic myocardial hypertrophy are progressive and lead to death, while others such as myocarditis improve but may cause residual abnormalities.

BACTERIAL ENDOCARDITIS

Bacterial endocarditis involves infection of the endocardium or of the endothelium of the great vessels. This condition usually occurs as a complication of congenital or rheumatic heart disease but occasionally develops without preexisting heart disease. Bacterial endocarditis is often divided into subacute and acute forms, the latter being of shorter duration, more commonly caused by a staphylococcus, and more frequently occurring without preexisting heart disease. This classification has limited use clinically because there is considerable overlap between acute and subacute types.

Streptococcus viridans is the most common causative agent; streptococcus faecalis and staphylococcus aureus occur less commonly. Rarely, other bacteria or fungi are involved. Bacterial endocarditis usually occurs in cardiac conditions where a pressure difference leads to a jet lesion. The congenital cardiac anomalies most often associated with endocarditis are ventricular septal defect, patent ductus arteriosus, aortic stenosis, and tetralogy of Fallot. Endocarditis can also occur in patients with aorticopulmonary shunts, such as a Blalock-Taussig shunt. It can involve the mitral or aortic valves in patients with rheumatic heart disease. Endocarditis is extremely rare in patients with atrial septal defect.

The cardiac lesions consist of vegetations of fibrin, leukocytes, platelets, and bacteria. Many clinical manifestations are related to destructive aspects of the infection or to embolization of portions of the vegetation. Endocarditis, particularly from staphylococcus, may cause valvular damage such as perforation of the aortic cusps or ruptured chordae tendinae of the mitral valve. Embolization may occur either in the pulmonary or the systemic circulation and cause infarction, abscess, or inflammation. Emboli to the lungs, kidneys, spleen, or brain are reported most frequently because in each location there are clinical or laboratory findings of the phenomenon.

Endocarditis occurs rarely before the age of 5 years. Fever, weight loss, anemia, and elevation of the erythrocyte sedimentation rate are common clinical findings in patients with bacterial endocarditis. The diagnosis should be suspected in any child with a significant cardiac murmur and a prolonged fever.

The appearance of a new murmur may indicate bacterial endocarditis, although a change in intensity of a murmur is not necessarily an indication of bacterial endocarditis. Congestive cardiac failure may develop.

Signs and symptoms of embolic phenomenon should be sought. Signs of recurrent pneumonia or a pleuritic type of pain may indicate embolization of infected material to the lungs. Signs of systemic embolization, such as splenomegaly, hematuria, splinter hemorrhages, and central nervous system signs, should be sought in any febrile patient with congenital cardiac disease. Half of the patients with bacterial endocarditis show findings of embolization.

The diagnosis can be confirmed by obtaining the organisms from a blood culture. Six blood cultures should be taken within the first 12 or 24 hours that endocarditis is suspected. It is not necessary to wait for a fever spike, since the chance of obtaining a positive culture is more dependent upon the volume of blood drawn.

If the patient is very ill or the clinical diagnosis typical, antibiotic treatment can be initiated immediately after the cultures are obtained and before the results of the culture are available. If the diagnosis is questionable, initiation of therapy should await the results of the blood cultures. Exact treatment depends upon the organism isolated and its antibiotic sensitivities. Usually, penicillin and streptomycin are the preferred antibiotics and are given in large dosages parenterally. Antibiotics may need to be changed if antibiotic sensitivities so indicate. Therapy is continued for 6 weeks. Following completion of therapy, blood cultures should be obtained to verify eradication of the infection.

Despite the availability of antibiotics, bacterial endocarditis can lead to major complications such as valvular damage or permanent sequelae resulting from embolization; occasionally, the disease is fatal.

Major efforts should be made to prevent the development of bacterial endocarditis in children with cardiac anomalies. The methods by which this can be accomplished are presented in Chapter 6 (*Management and Treatment*).

MARFAN'S SYNDROME

Marfan's syndrome is an autosomal dominant disease affecting connective tissue and leading to characteristic physical findings and cardiac lesions. These patients are tall and thin, showing a high incidence of kyphoscoliosis, pectus carinatum, arachnodactyly, high-arched palate, and loose joints. Dislocation of the lens is common.

Cardiac anomalies occur in almost all patients and lead to premature death, although death rarely occurs in childhood. Aneurysmal dilatation of the ascending aorta and aortic sinuses occurs and leads to aortic regurgitation. The degree of aortic insufficiency may become severe. Dissecting aneurysms can develop in the ascending aorta and lead to death. Mitral insufficiency and prolapse of the valve cusps are also common, resulting from elongated chordae tendinae.

Many children with Marfan's syndrome are asymptomatic, but severe aortic or mitral regurgitation requires valve replacement. Replacement of the aortic valve is often combined with replacement of the ascending aorta with a Dacron graft in order to prevent dissecting aneurysm. The long-term prognosis following these operations is yet to be determined.

PROLAPSING MITRAL VALVE

This condition has been described with increasing frequency in the last decade. It occurs predominately in females, and is usually first recognized in adolescence. There may be a positive family history, but the etiology and pathology are largely unknown. Echocardiographic and angiocardiographic studies have given information suggesting that in this condition the posterior and occasionally the anterior mitral valve cusp prolapse into the left atrium. The prolapse occurs maximally in midsystole and may be associated with mitral regurgitation beginning in mid or late systole.

The auscultatory findings are diagnostic. At the apex there is a mid or late blowing systolic murmur that often begins with one or multiple midsystolic clicks. The characteristics of the murmur are variable. Any maneuver that decreases left ventricular diastolic volume, such as a Valsalva maneuver, standing, or inhalation of amyl nitrate, causes the murmur to begin earlier, last longer, and become louder.

The prognosis is good for patients with prolapsing mitral valve, but long-term follow-up studies are needed. An electrocardiogram should be performed periodically to identify ST segment and T wave changes and prolongation of the QT interval. Patients with such alterations are reported to be at a higher risk for arrhythmias followed by sudden death, but the exact incidence of this is unknown. Bacterial endocarditis may occur in individuals with mitral valve prolapse; individuals with mitral insufficiency should receive prophylactic antibiotics at times of predictable risk of bacteremia.

PERICARDITIS

Pericarditis can result from several disease entities. The most common in my experience are: 1) idiopathic, presumed viral; 2) purulent; 3) rheumatoid arthritis; 4) uremia; and 5) neoplastic diseases.

In these conditions, both the pericardial sac and the visceral pericardium are involved. As a result of the inflammation, fluid may accumulate within the sac. The symptoms that result from pericardial fluid depend upon the status of the myocardium and the volume and the speed at which the fluid accumulates. A slow accumulation of a large volume is often better tolerated than the rapid accumulation of a small volume.

Cardiac tamponade can develop because of fluid accumulation within the pericardial sac. The pericardial fluid can compress the heart and can interfere with ventricular filling. Three mechanisms compensate for the tamponade: 1) elevation of atrial and ventricular end-diastolic pressures; 2) tachycardia to compensate for lowered stroke volume; and 3) increased diastolic blood pressure from peripheral vasoconstriction to compensate for diminished cardiac output.

Clinical and Laboratory Findings

The clinical and laboratory findings are related to: 1) the inflammation of the pericardium, 2) cardiac tamponade, and 3) etiologic factors.

Pericarditis is accompanied by pain in about half the patients. This may be dull, sharp, or stabbing. The pain may be located in the left thorax, neck, or shoulder and is improved when the patient is sitting. A pericardial friction rub, a rough scratchy sound, may be present over the precordium. It is louder when the patient is sitting, when the examiner uses the bell of the stethoscope, or when the stethoscope is pressed against the chest wall. The rub is evanescent, so repeated examinations may be needed to identify it. There is no direct relationship between the amount of pericardial fluid and the presence of a rub, but large effusions may not demonstrate a rub.

Electrocardiographic Features

The electrocardiogram usually shows ST segment and T wave changes. Early in the course of the disease the ST segment is elevated and the T wave is upright. Subsequently, the ST segments return to the isoelectric line and the T waves become diffusely inverted. Later, both ST segments and T waves return to normal. The QRS voltage may be reduced, particularly with large fluid accumulations.

Roentgenographic Features

The thoracic roentgenogram may be normal, but an enlarged cardiac silhouette develops with accumulation of pericardial fluid.

Cardiac tamponade is reflected by several physical findings. The patient may appear in distress and be more comfortable when sitting. The neck veins are distended and, in contrast to normal, are increased on inspiration. The heart sounds may be muffled. Hepatomegaly may be found. Tachycardia develops and is a valuable means of following the patient. As the stroke volume falls because of the tamponade, the heart rate increases to maintain cardiac output. The pulse pressure also narrows, and this can also be measured accurately and in a serial manner to follow the patient's course. Pulsus paradoxus, a decrease in pulse pressure of more than 20 mm Hg with inspiration, is also highly diagnostic of tamponade and can often be identified by palpation of the radial pulse.

Historical and physical findings may suggest an etiology of the pericardial effusion such as a history of neoplasm or uremia. In many patients, no etiology is found for acute pericarditis. Certain viral agents such as Coxsackie B have been identified as causative agents for pericarditis. In these patients there is frequently a history of a preceding respiratory infection. Among patients with purulent pericarditis, Hemophilus influenzae and pneumococcus are the most common organisms. Purulent pericarditis usually occurs in infancy and may follow or be associated with infection at another site, such as pneumonia or osteomyelitis. The infants often show a high leukocyte count and appear to be very septic.

Pericarditis can develop secondary to rheumatoid arthritis and may occur before other manifestations of this disease. Usually children show high fever, leukocytosis, and other systemic signs. Tamponade rarely occurs.

Pericardial effusion can be recognized quite accurately by echocardiography, and this technique may be helpful in diagnosing suspicious cases.

Treatment

Pericardiocentesis is indicated in many patients to confirm the diagnosis, identify the etiology, or treat pericardial tamponade. In patients with purulent pericarditis, pericardiocentesis is indicated, since reaching an etiologic diagnosis is imperative so that appropriate antibiotic therapy can be initiated. Other than in patients with neoplasm and purulent pericarditis, the analysis of the fluid rarely yields a diagnosis.

Pericardiocentesis is indicated often as an emergency procedure to treat the cardiac tamponade by removing fluid and thereby allowing adequate cardiac filling. At times, particularly with recurrent tamponade, a thoracotomy with creation of a pericardial window is indicated to decompress the pericardial sac.

Other treatment may be indicated for pericarditis. Symptomatic relief of pain is indicated. Digitalis and diuretics are contraindicated because they slow the heart rate and reduce the filling pressure (as against the normal compensatory mechanisms). High dosages of antibiotics are indicated in purulent pericarditis, the type to be determined by antibiotic sensitivities, and open or closed drainage may be necessary.

CARDIAC ARRHYTHMIAS

Disturbance of cardiac rate and conduction may occur in children, without preceding cardiac disease, as a manifestation of congenital or acquired cardiac disease or as a complication of drug therapy, particularly of digitalis therapy.

Cardiac arrhythmias can be generally classified as: 1) alterations in cardiac pacemaker activity, or 2) abnormalities of conduction.

Pacemaker Disturbances

Cardiac arrhythmias result from alterations in the rate of discharge of pacemakers at the atrial, junctional, or ventricular level.

Atrial Arrhythmias

Sinus Arrhythmia (Fig. 51).   This is a variation of normal sinus rhythm. It describes the normal increase in cardiac rate with inspiration and the slowing with expiration. Sometimes with expiration, nodal escape occurs.

Premature Atrial Systole.   This occurs uncommonly in children and arises from an ectopic atrial focus. On the electrocardiogram it is recognized by a P wave that has an abnormal shape and occurs earlier than normal (Fig. 52). There is no compensatory pause. No treatment is required.

Sinus Tachycardia.   The normal sinoatrial node may discharge at a rapid rate of up to 210 beats per minute. This occurs not because of an ectopic pacemaker but in response to some stimulus or as a reflex response. Fever, shock, atropine, and epinephrine are among the causes of sinus tachycardia. The increased heart rate does not require treatment, but the tachycardia should be considered a clinical finding that requires diagnosis and perhaps treatment.

Paroxysmal Supraventricular Tachycardia.   Paroxysmal supraventricular tachycardia, although infrequent in children, is important because it may lead to death if untreated. In pediatric patients, this arrhythmia occurs predominately in boys and in the neonatal period. Typically, a previously healthy child develops poor feeding, sweating, irritability, and rapid respiration. If the arrhythmia is unrecognized and untreated, congestive cardiac failure may progress until death occurs in 2 to 3 days. Arrhythmia is not difficult to recognize when examining the heart. A heart rate of 250 to 350 per minute (Fig. 53) is found and is remarkably regular, showing no variation as the child breathes, cries, or becomes quiet. Digitalization (see below) converts the tachycardia to a normal sinus rhythm within hours following the first dose and should be maintained for 6 months.

The prognosis is excellent because in the majority of infants no underlying cardiac malformation is present and recurrent episodes are rare. However, a few infants with either Ebstein's malformation or Wolff-Parkinson-White syndrome will have repeated episodes of supraventricular tachycardia.

Atrial Flutter.   In atrial flutter, the atrial rate may be between 280 and 400 per minute, and there is a 2 : 1 or greater degree of block so that ventricular rate is slower than the atrial rate (Fig. 54). On the electrocardiogram the atrial activity appears not as distinct P waves, but rather it has a saw-tooth

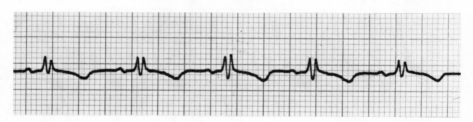

Figure 51.   Electrocardiographic tracing of sinus arrhythmia. Each QRS complex is preceded by a P wave, but interval between each P wave is variable.

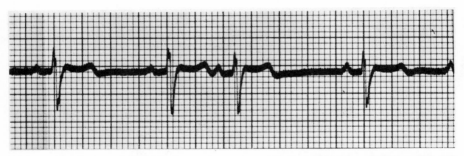

Figure 52. Electrocardiographic tracing showing premature atrial contraction. Third P wave from left occurs early. No compensatory pause.

appearance. This arrhythmia can occur in infants without an underlying condition or in children with conditions such as endocardial fibroelastosis, Ebstein's malformation, or rheumatic mitral disease that lead to a greatly enlarged atrium. Digitalization or cardioversion with a very small wattage converts the rhythm to a sinus mechanism.

Atrial Fibrillation. Atrial fibrillation is associated with a rate of atrial depolarization greater than 400 per minute, so atrial activity is chaotic. Distinct P waves are not seen, but atrial activity is evident as small, irregular wave forms on the electrocardiogram (Fig. 55). Ventricular response is irregular. This arrhythmia also results from conditions that chronically dilate the atria. Digitalis is indicated to slow the ventricular response. Cardioversion is usually unsuccessful and requires a high wattage.

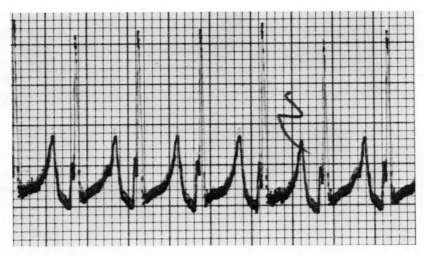

Figure 53. Electrocardiographic tracing of paroxysmal supraventricular tachycardia.

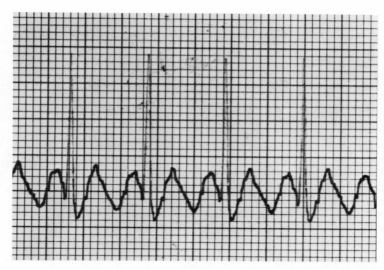

Figure 54. Electrocardiographic tracing of atrial flutter. Two P waves occur for every QRS complex.

Junctional Arrhythmias

Ectopic arrhythmias can arise from the atrioventricular node and are called nodal or junctional premature beats, or tachycardia. The QRS complex is normal. The P waves may appear shortly before the QRS complex and be abnormal in form, be buried within the QRS complex, or follow the QRS complex. The rate of junctional tachycardia is often around 200 per minute and requires digitalization.

Ventricular Arrhythmias

Ventricular arrhythmias arise from ectopic foci in the His bundles and are characterized by widened QRS complexes and abnormal T waves.

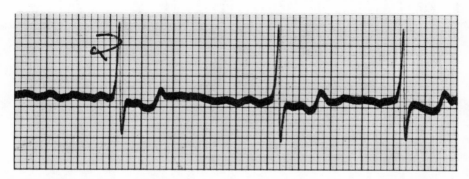

Figure 55. Electrocardiographic tracing of atrial fibrillation. Wavy isoelectric line reflects the irregular and rapid atrial activity.

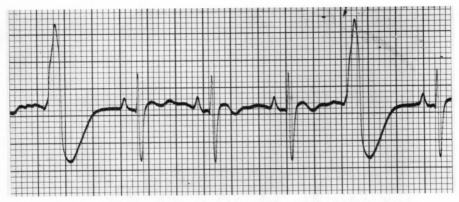

Figure 56. Electrocardiographic tracing of premature ventricular contractions. These ectopic beats noted as widened QRS complexes associated with abnormal T waves.

Ventricular Premature Beats. In children, premature ventricular contractions are usually benign arrhythmias. They are recognized by bizarre QRS complexes falling irregularly in the normal cardiac rhythm (Fig. 56). The QRS is widened, has a different configuration from the normal QRS complex, does not follow a P wave, and is associated with a large T wave. There is a compensatory pause following the ectopic beat. Generally, premature ventricular contractions are unifocal, meaning that each of the aberrant QRS complexes has an identical configuration. Occasionally, multifocal premature ventricular contractions are present, leading to QRS complexes with varying contours. Without treatment the prognosis is excel-

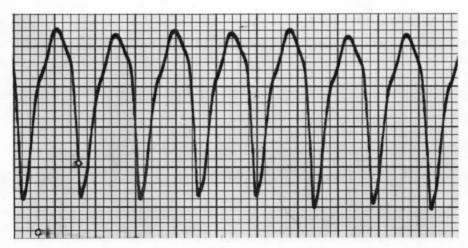

Figure 57. Electrocardiographic tracing of ventricular tachycardia. Widened QRS complexes occurring at regular intervals without evidence of atrial activity.

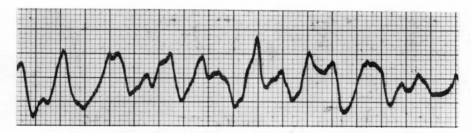

Figure 58. Electrocardiographic tracing of ventricular fibrillation. Irregular disorganized ventricular activity.

lent in unifocal premature ventricular contractions; whereas multifocal premature ventricular contractions are often related to myocardial disease. They may even develop as a sign of digitalis toxicity and require the discontinuance of that medication and careful monitoring. Premature ventricular contractions in children usually require no treatment.

Ventricular Tachycardia. Ventricular tachycardia arises as a rapidly discharging ventricular focus at a rate of 150-250 per minute. These are usually serious arrhythmias that are associated with symptoms of chest pain, palpitations, or syncope. This rhythm may occur in normal children as a manifestation of digitalis toxicity in myocarditis or as a terminal event. The electrocardiogram shows wide bizarre QRS complexes and often P waves occurring at a slower rate (Fig. 57). Ventricular tachycardia requires immediate treatment with propranolol, procainamide, or lidocaine or, at times, cardioversion.

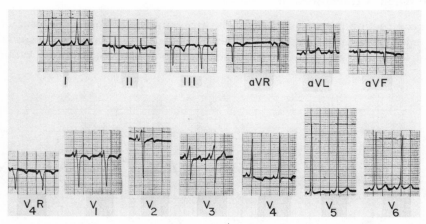

Figure 59. Electrocardiogram showing Wolff-Parkinson-White (WPW) syndrome. PR interval is shortened and QRS complex is broadened. Delta wave, indicated by slurred initial portion of QRS complex, particularly noted in leads I and V_6.

175

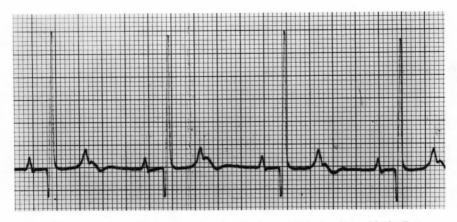

Figure 60. Electrocardiographic tracing showing second degree heart block. Every second P wave is followed by a QRS complex.

Ventricular Fibrillation. The electrocardiographic finding of ventricular fibrillation often represents a terminal event and is seen as wide, bizarre, irregularly occurring wave forms of various amplitudes (Fig. 58). Cardiac output is markedly decreased. It is treated by the methods outlined in the subsequent section on cardiopulmonary arrest.

Conduction Disturbances

Most major conduction disturbances occur between the atrium and the ventricles at the level of the atrioventricular node.

Shortened Atrioventricular Conduction

The conduction through or around the atrioventricular node may be accelerated, and such patients tend to develop episodes of paroxysmal supraventricular tachycardia. One of these conditions, the preexcitation Wolff-

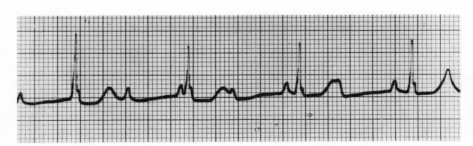

Figure 61. Electrocardiographic tracing showing complete heart block. P waves and QRS complexes are occurring independently and the ventricular rate is slow.

Parkinson-White syndrome, has three components: 1) a shortened PR interval, 2) a widened QRS complex, and 3) a delta wave—slowly inscribed initial portion of the QRS complex (Fig. 59). Wolff-Parkinson-White syndrome may be present in patients without other cardiac anomalies and in patients with Ebstein's malformation. In the other form the PR interval is short, but the QRS is of normal duration.

Prolonged Atrioventricular Conduction

Several forms of prolonged atrioventricular conduction have been described.

First Degree Heart Block. This is represented by prolongation of the PR interval beyond the normal range, and each P wave is followed by a QRS complex. Digitalis, acute rheumatic fever, and acute infections are causes of first degree heart block. It does not require treatment.

Second Degree Heart Block. In this form, each P wave is not followed by a QRS complex. There may be a 2:1 or 3:1 block between the atria and the ventricles (Fig. 60). Treatment is not indicated unless there are syncopal episodes, and then a pacemaker should be placed.

Third Degree Heart Block. This is complete atrioventricular block. There is dissociation between the atria and the ventricles, and the atrial impulse does not influence the ventricles (Fig. 61). The ventricular rate is slow, and therefore its stroke volume is increased, leading to soft systolic and diastolic murmurs and cardiomegaly.

Third degree heart block can occur congenitally and generally has a good prognosis except in those cases with a family history of heart block. It may also develop from digitalis toxicity and following cardiac surgery. The prognosis for recovery from the latter is poor. Complete heart block may be associated with syncopal episodes (Stokes-Adams attacks), and usually not with congestive cardiac failure, unless there are additional cardiac disorders.

If the heart rate is persistently low, less than 40 per minute, or syncopal episodes occur, a permanently implanted pacemaker is indicated. A pacemaker is indicated in all children with postoperative heart block because of the high incidence of sudden death. It is wise to wait a month after operation before implanting a permanent pacemaker, as within that time sinus rhythm may return.

5

CARDIAC CONDITIONS
IN THE NEONATE

NEONATAL PHYSIOLOGY

Not only in newborn infants with congenital cardiac disease, but also among those with pulmonary disease or other serious illnesses, the distinctive and transitional features of the neonatal circulation may lead to cardiopulmonary abnormalities. Understanding the anatomic and physiologic features of the transition from fetal to adult circulation will aid the physician in caring for critically ill neonates.

The fetal circulation differs from that of the postnatal state. In the fetus the pulmonary and systemic circulations are parallel, rather than in series. In the fetal circulation, both ventricles eject blood into the aorta and receive systemic venous return. The right ventricle ejects a greater volume than the left ventricle. Postnatally, the circulation is different in that the ventricles and the circulation are in series. The right ventricle receives the systemic venous return, and the left ventricle alone ejects blood into the aorta. Left ventricular and right ventricular outputs are equal. The transition from a parallel to a series circulation normally occurs at birth, but in distressed neonates the parallel circulation may persist and the evolution to series circulation be delayed.

The fetal circulation also has three distinctive anatomic structures: the placenta, the patent ductus arteriosus, and the patent foramen ovale. The blood returning to the fetus from the placenta enters the right atrium and flows predominantly from the right to the left atrium through the patent foramen ovale (Fig. 62). This stream passes to the left ventricle and the ascending aorta, supplying the head with the proper level of oxygenated blood. The blood that returns from the head returns to the heart in the

178

superior vena cava and flows principally into the right ventricle. Right ventricular output passes into the pulmonary trunk, and the major portion (85 percent) flows through the ductus into the aorta, while a smaller amount (15 percent) flows into the lungs.

The major factor influencing the pattern and distribution of fetal blood flow is the relative vascular resistance of the pulmonary and systemic circuits. In the fetus, in contrast to the adult, the pulmonary vascular resistance is very elevated and the systemic vascular resistance is low. Prenatally, the pulmonary arterioles possess a thick medial coat and a narrowed lumen. These anatomic features of the pulmonary arterioles are accentuated by the relative hypoxic environment of the fetus, hypoxia being a potent stimulus for pulmonary vasoconstriction. The systemic vascular resistance is unusually low, primarily because of the large flow through the placenta, which has low resistance. In the fetus the pulmonary

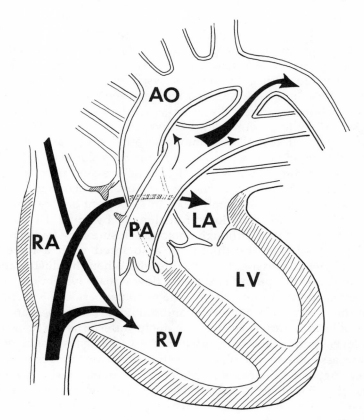

Figure 62. Central circulation in the fetus. Predominant flow from inferior vena cava is through the patent foramen ovale into the left atrium. Major portion of right ventricular flow is through the patent ductus arteriosus. Ao = aorta. LA = left atrium. LV = left ventricle. PA = pulmonary artery. RA = right atrium. RV = right ventricle.

179

vascular resistance is five times greater than the systemic vascular resistance, the reverse of the adult circulation.

Because the systolic pressures in both ventricles and great vessels are identical, the distribution of blood flow depends upon the relative vascular resistances. As a result, a relatively small volume of blood flows through the lungs, and a large volume passes through the ductus from right to left into the aorta. A considerable portion of the combined ventricular output flows through the placenta.

The right-to-left shunt at the atrial level in the fetus depends in part upon the streaming effect caused by the position of the valve of the foramen ovale. This ridge tends to divert blood from the inferior vena cava through the defect into the left atrium. Since the atrial pressures are identical, the shunt also depends on the relative compliances of the ventricles. About one third of the total flow returning to the right atrium crosses the foramen ovale.

At birth the distinctive features of the circulation and the vascular resistances are suddenly changed. A major reversal of resistance occurs because of the separation of the placenta and the onset of respiration. The loss of the placenta, which has acted essentially as an arteriovenous fistula, is associated with a doubling of systemic vascular resistance. The expansion of the lungs is associated with a sevenfold drop in pulmonary vascular resistance, principally from vasodilatation of pulmonary arterioles secondary to a normal level of oxygen in inspired air.

Coincidental with the fall in pulmonary vascular resistance, the volume of pulmonary blood flow increases, and thus the volume of blood returning to the left atrium increases. The left atrial pressure rises, exceeds the right atrial pressure, and closes the foramen ovale functionally. Anatomically, the atrial septum ultimately seals in 75 percent of children.

The ductus narrows and closes functionally by muscular contraction within 24 hours of birth, although anatomic closure may be delayed for a week. The closure of the ductus is associated with a lowering of pulmonary arterial pressure to normal levels. When the ductus and foramen ovale close, the pulmonary blood flow equals systemic blood flow and the circulations are in series. In the neonatal period the changes that occur in the ductus, foramen ovale, and pulmonary arterioles are reversible. The pulmonary arterioles and the ductus arteriosus are responsive to oxygen levels and acidosis. Increase in the vascular resistance occurs in conditions associated with hypoxia. Although minor changes occur at pO_2 of 50 mm Hg, large increases in pulmonary vascular resistance occur at pO_2 less than 25 mm Hg. If acidosis coexists with hypoxia, the increase in pulmonary resistance is far greater than at comparable levels of pO_2 occurring at normal pH.

Neonates with pulmonary parenchymal disease, such as respiratory distress syndrome, therefore develop increased pulmonary vascular resistance and increased pulmonary arterial pressure because of hypoxia. If acidosis complicates the illness, the changes are even greater. Subsequent to elevation of right ventricular pressure, right atrial pressure increases, opening the foramen ovale and causing a right-to-left shunt.

In a similar way the ductus arteriosus of a neonate is also responsive to oxygen. With hypoxia, the ductus may reopen, and should the pulmonary resistance be simultaneously elevated, a right-to-left shunt could occur through the ductus arteriosus. Thus, cyanosis in the neonate with pulmonary parenchymal disease can result from right-to-left shunting of blood, as well as from pulmonary diffusion defects. Administration of 100 percent oxygen may correct both of these abnormalities, but the improvement is often not sufficient to exclude the diagnosis of cyanotic forms of congenital cardiac disease. Oxygen administration to cyanotic patients with congenital cardiac disease may also lessen the degree of cyanosis.

CARDIAC DISEASE IN THE NEWBORN

Congenital cardiac malformations may lead to severe cardiac symptoms and death in the neonatal period. The types of cardiac malformations causing symptoms in this age group are generally different from those leading to symptoms later in infancy. Among the latter group, symptoms usually depend upon a large volume of pulmonary blood flow, such as in ventricular septal defect, in which congestive failure develops at about 6 weeks of age. Other conditions, such as tetralogy of Fallot, await the development of sufficient stenosis before becoming symptomatic. In the neonate, *congestive cardiac failure* and *hypoxia* are the major cardiac symptom complexes.

Congestive cardiac failure in the neonatal period results most commonly from: 1) anomalies causing outflow obstruction, particularly to the left side of the heart, and which are often associated with a hypoplastic ventricle; 2) volume overload from an insufficient cardiac valve; or 3) systemic arteriovenous fistula. Rarely in the neonatal period do cardiac conditions with left-to-right shunts place large volumes upon the ventricles and lead to symptoms. Occasionally, in prematurely born infants, a patent ductus arteriosus may lead to signs of cardiac failure. Presumably, the pulmonary vasculature approaches normal levels more quickly than in full-term infants. The resultant large volume of pulmonary blood flow causes overload of the left ventricle.

Hypoplastic left ventricle syndrome is the most frequent cause of cardiac failure in this age group (Fig. 63). The term hypoplastic left ventricle encompasses several cardiac malformations, each associated with a diminutive left ventricle and with similar clinical and physiologic features; included are aortic atresia, mitral atresia, and severe aortic stenosis. In each, severe obstruction is present to both left ventricular inflow and

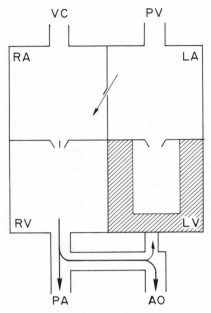

Figure 63. Central circulation in aortic atresia.

outflow. Whether from an atretic mitral valve or a small left ventricle, filling of the left ventricle is impeded. The left atrial pressure elevates, forcing the foramen ovale to herniate and thereby permitting a small amount of blood to flow from the left to the right atrium. The volume of shunt is not sufficient to decompress the left atrium, so the pressure in this chamber rises and leads to elevation of pulmonary capillary pressure and ultimately to pulmonary edema. Left ventricular outflow is also severely obstructed.

Patent ductus arteriosus is a major component of each abnormality classed as hypoplastic left ventricle syndrome. The flow through the ductus is from right to left and represents the major source of systemic arterial blood. In fact, the left ventricular output may be absent, or so small that the flow into the ascending aorta and to the coronary arteries is in a retrograde direction via the ductus arteriosus. Coarctation of the aorta may complicate the anatomic features.

These patients show severe congestive cardiac failure and low cardiac output in the first week of life. The peripheral pulses are weak, and the skin is mottled because of poor tissue perfusion. A soft, nonspecific murmur may be heard but often no murmur is found. The electrocardiogram appears normal for the age. Thoracic roentgenograms show an enlarged heart and accentuated pulmonary arterial and venous markings. Death

182

usually occurs in the first week of life. Corrective or palliative operations are not available for infants with hypoplastic left ventricle syndrome.

Coarctation of the aorta, either isolated or coexisting with other cardiac malformations, is the other common cause of congestive cardiac failure in the neonate. Clinical diagnosis may be difficult because the low cardiac output from congestive failure minimizes the blood pressure difference between the arms and legs. Following treatment with digitalis, a blood pressure differential may develop as the cardiac output increases. Cardiomegaly and an electrocardiographic pattern of right ventricular hypertrophy and inverted ST segment and T waves in the left precordium are found. Much less frequently, aortic and pulmonary stenosis may lead to congestive cardiac failure early in life.

Volume overload placed on either ventricle may lead to neonatal cardiac failure. The most common, systemic arteriovenous fistula, as occurring in the great vein of Galen, results in a high output failure. The arteriovenous fistula is associated with low systemic arterial resistance and an increased volume of blood flow through the shunt. The increased flow through the right side of the heart leads to profound cardiac symptoms early in life. Prior to birth, cardiac failure is absent because of the low systemic vascular resistance prenatally. With the loss of the placenta, systemic resistance increases and volume shunted through the fistula increases. An arteriovenous fistula may be recognized by auscultation for a continuous murmur over the heart or liver or other peripheral sites. Operative obliteration of the fistula, if possible, is curative.

Insufficiency of cardiac valves is an uncommon cause of neonatal cardiac failure.

Severe cardiac symptoms also occur in the neonatal period because of *hypoxia* due to inadequate mixing, as occurs in complete transposition of the great arteries with intact ventricular septum. Severe hypoxia can also occur in conditions with severe obstruction to pulmonary blood flow and an intracardiac shunt. In the neonate, tetralogy of Fallot, often with pulmonary atresia; pulmonary atresia with hypoplastic right ventricle; and tricuspid atresia are the conditions that lead to this state. Neonates with hypoxia show extreme cyanosis and rapid, difficult respirations. Acidosis can develop quickly because of the hypoxia; cardiac failure is usually not a major problem. Administration of oxygen is usually of little benefit. Neonates with complete transposition of the great arteries require a Rashkind septostomy or an operation such as a Blalock-Hanlon procedure to improve intracardiac mixing, and those with inadequate pulmonary blood flow require an aorticopulmonary shunt to improve oxygenation.

Thus, it can be seen that a diverse group of cardiac conditions causes symptoms in early infancy. Some, such as tetralogy of Fallot or coarctation of the aorta, can be corrected or palliated by operation. For those with transposed great arteries, cardiac catheterization with performance of a Rashkind balloon atrial septostomy is lifesaving. For others, such as those with aortic atresia, no procedure is available presently. Because of the potential for correction or palliation, any neonate with severe cardiac symptoms should be studied by cardiac catheterization and angiocardiography to define the anatomic details of the cardiac malformation. Although some risk (3 percent mortality) is involved in the performance of cardiac catheterization in neonates, it is outweighed by the likelihood of finding a treatable form of cardiac disease. Following definition of the malformation, appropriate decisions can be made concerning further therapy.

An aggressive diagnostic and therapeutic approach is warranted in neonates. This approach begins with the prompt recognition of cardiac disease in the newborn nursery. Treatment of the cardiac symptoms should be initiated, and the infant should be immediately referred to a cardiac center for definitive diagnosis and therapy.

6

MANAGEMENT AND TREATMENT

GENERAL CONSIDERATIONS

Optimum care of the child with congenital cardiac disease entails attention to the effect of the disease upon the behavioral, psychological, and intellectual growth of the child, and upon the family. Other considerations are the proper definition of the disease and the medical and surgical management. In this age of sophisticated diagnostic and surgical procedures, the common psychological factors of chronic disease are frequently overlooked.

Some patients undergo expensive and extensive surgical procedures to correct their cardiac malformations, but are "crippled" by the severe emotional problems of many children with chronic disease. Because of a murmur or cardiac disease, many potential problems may develop in the family. It is of the utmost importance that the physician recognize these problems.

On the initial visit, following the review of the clinical and laboratory findings with the parents, they should be given ample opportunity to express their feelings and to ask questions. It is wise to listen and to reassure them. A feeling of guilt, although seldom expressed, is often present. In explaining cardiac defects, I have found it helpful to point out that, except for the cases due to rubella and mumps viral infections, we know of few causes of congenital cardiac disease. If there were something that mothers were doing wrong, it would be common knowledge.

Many parents, because of feelings of guilt or sympathy, assume an overprotective and solicitous attitude toward the child with cardiac disease; this may, in part, be fostered by the physician's attitudes. *Unless there are contraindications,* the child should be treated the same as his siblings in chores, responsibilities, and punishment. He should partake as fully as possible in family activities. Family life should not center in the cardiac patient. It is important also to stress the emotional needs of other children in the family. Whenever possible, the affected child should attend regular school. Grandparents in particular must be cautioned of the dangers of an overly sympathetic or solicitous approach.

In summary, *the child must be treated like other children to the fullest possible extent.*

Family Counseling

Following the discovery of congenital cardiac disease in one of their children, parents are often concerned about the risks of having a second child similarly affected. If, in the proband, congenital cardiac disease is not part of a recognized syndrome and there is no previous family history of congenital cardiac anomalies, the risk of a second affected child is probably twice that of the first. The incidence of congenital cardiac disease in the population is 0.7 percent, reflecting an incidence of 1/135. If a second child in a family is affected, the form of cardiac disease will probably be the same or similar. There are families in which several members of one generation show the same form of congenital cardiac disease. Interestingly, one exception seems to be complete transposition of the great vessels, where the occurrence of multiple, or even two, instances in a family is rare.

If a second child does have cardiac disease, the risk of a subsequent child also having cardiac disease is even higher.

If the child shows one of the recognizable syndromes associated with cardiac disease, specific family counseling should be given. It is not the physician's responsibility to instruct the parents about whether they should or should not attempt to have more children, but he should advise them of the available information so that they can reach a rational decision.

For the following conditions, the mode of inheritance and risk of another affected child are given.

Turner's syndrome	Negligibly small
Down's syndrome	Less than 1 percent for nondisjunction type; 5 to 20 percent for translocation type
Trisomy 13	If parent is a carrier, 10 percent
Trisomy 18	Probably no greater than 2 to 3 percent
Marfan's syndrome	If parent is affected, 50 percent; otherwise not increased
Rubella	None
Idiopathic hypercalcemia	Unknown

For any child with a congenital cardiac anomaly, the physician must make recommendations or answer questions about four general areas: exercise, diet, frequency of follow-up visits, and bacterial endocarditis prophylaxis.

Exercise Limitations

Most children with congenital cardiac anomalies can be allowed a normal range of physical activity; they should realize that the anomaly may limit their ability to exercise. The child should be permitted to participate in physical education in school. Teachers must understand that the child may have to stop and rest sooner than the other children. In addition, the child should not be pushed to extremes of physical activity or to perform in unfavorable situations such as extreme heat or cold.

Children with moderate or severe aortic stenosis should be excluded from competitive athletics; exertion can be fatal in these children.

In the presence of an active inflammatory disease involving the myocardium, such as acute rheumatic carditis or myocarditis, the child should be placed on modified bed rest. Complete bed rest is difficult to achieve because of a child's natural activeness. As an alternative, children can spend most of their time sitting, or lying on the couch, and can be allowed up to the bathroom and dinner table. Television helps to keep children entertained.

Children with congenital cardiac anomalies may be inappropriately restricted by school authorities, even when the school has been informed that there is no need for exercise restriction. This reflects an unrealistic fear that teachers sometimes have about children with cardiac disease, a fear that arises from ignorance of congenital cardiac anomalies and the association of all cardiac disease with heart attacks and sudden death. In any correspondence regarding a child with congenital cardiac disease, whether to a referring physician or to a school, the recommended level of exercise should be clearly defined.

Following pediatric cardiac operations, the level of exercise can be gradually increased to full participation 4 to 6 weeks postoperatively, provided no major complication such as congestive cardiac failure is present. After recovery from this operation, the child should be permitted normal activity as tolerated.

Diet

Most children with cardiac anomalies do not require a special diet, except for those with cardiac failure in whom a low sodium diet is indicated. Infants are given the standard milk preparations for prematures that contain about 7 mEq/L of sodium. In older children, salt restriction varies from recommendation of no added salt and avoidance of foods with high salt content, such as potato chips, French fries, hot dogs, and luncheon meat, to a modified diet limiting sodium.

Children with congenital cardiac anomalies may be small in stature because of the effect of the defect upon the circulation or because of problems coexisting with the anomaly. In symptomatic infants the problem may be aggravated because, since they fatigue on eating, their caloric intake is limited.

Between the ages of 1 and 4 years, the appetite of many children is considered poor by their parents. The parents of healthy children in this age range often complain about their child's eating habits. Normally children at this age eat one "good" meal a day and the rest of the time pick at their food. They may be food faddists, and because they are small, do not eat adult portions of food. The rate of weight gain compared to the first year of life markedly decreases at about 1 year of age and the child gains only about 4 pounds a year, in contrast to the expected gain of 14 pounds during the first year of life.

Each of these factors leads to concern in many parents, and these concerns are increased in the parents of children with congenital cardiac anomalies who are small. They believe that if the child would only eat, he would grow. This leads to turmoil, unpleasant meals, and frustration. These problems can be reduced by anticipatory guidance in discussing with the parents what they should expect as their child enters the period of 1 to 4 years of age. Many families with children with congenital cardiac disease (as well as those with normal children) can be helped by such counseling.

Follow-Up Care

Most children with cardiac anomalies require periodic evaluation. The reasons for the evaluation and the type of information sought depend in large part upon the natural history of the cardiac condition. For instance, in a patient with a large ventricular septal defect, evidence of the development of pulmonary hypertension or congestive cardiac failure would be sought, while in aortic stenosis, evidence of left ventricular strain would be looked for. Thus, the frequency of return visits and the type of diagnostic studies performed on the patient's return are dictated by the symptoms and the natural history of the defect.

Usually infants are evaluated more frequently than older children because changes in circulation take place more rapidly in the first year of life.

Children with cardiac anomalies also require routine pediatric care. In infants with cardiac failure or other major symptoms, it is easy to overlook or fail to administer, because of illness, the routine immunizations, but these are an important component of the health care.

Bacterial Endocarditis Prophylaxis

Children with most forms of congenital cardiac anomalies and those with acquired valvular anomalies are at an increased risk for the development of bacterial endocarditis. The only exception is atrial septal defect, where bacterial endocarditis is rare. The potential for bacterial endocarditis exists whenever bacteremia occurs. While it is not possible to prevent bacteremia, it is possible to provide prophylaxis during certain types of operations or procedures when bacteremia could occur.

Operative or manipulative procedures involving the mouth or oropharynx, or the gastrointestinal or genitourinary tract, may be associated with bacteremia. Studies have shown that the administration of antibiotics within 1 hour prior to the procedure reduces the incidence of positive blood cultures. Thus, the American Heart Association has developed recommendations for antibiotic prophylaxis for procedures where a risk of bacteremia is present. These recommendations are listed below.

RECOMMENDATIONS FOR ANTIBIOTIC PROPHYLAXIS

For Dental Procedures and Tonsillectomy, Adenoidectomy and Bronchoscopy

For most patients:
  Penicillin
    Intramuscular:
      600,000 units of procaine penicillin G mixed with 200,000 units of crystalline penicillin G 1 hour prior to procedure and once daily for 2 days* following the procedure, or
    Oral:
      500 mg of penicillin V or phenethicillin 1 hour prior to procedure and then 250 mg every 6 hours for the remainder of that day and for the 2 days* following the procedure, or
      1,200,000 units of penicillin G 1 hour prior to procedure and then 600,000 units every 6 hours for the remainder of that day and for 2 days* following the procedure.
For patients suspected to be allergic to penicillin and for those on continual *oral* penicillin for rheumatic fever prophylaxis, who may harbor penicillin-resistant viridans streptococci:
  Erythromycin
    Oral:
      Adults: 500 mg 1½ to 2 hours prior to procedure and then 250 mg every 6 hours for the remainder of that day and for 2 days* following the procedure.

* or longer in the case of delayed healing

Children: 20 mg/kg orally 1½ to 2 hours prior to the procedure and then 10 mg/kg every 6 hours for the remainder of that day and for 2 days* following the procedure.

NOTE: Erythromycin preparations for parenteral use are also available.

For Gastrointestinal and Genitourinary Tract Surgery and Instrumentation, and Surgery of Infected Tissues

For most patients:

Penicillin

600,000 units of procaine penicillin G mixed with 200,000 units of crystalline penicillin G intramuscularly 1 hour prior to procedure and once daily for 2 days following the procedure.

plus

Streptomycin

1 to 2 gm intramuscularly, 1 hour prior to procedure and once daily for 2 days following the procedure.

Children: 40 mg/kg intramuscularly 1 hour prior to the procedure and once daily for 2 days following the procedure (not to exceed 1 gm/24 hours).

OR

Ampicillin

25 to 50 mg/kg orally or intravenously 1 hour prior to procedure and then 25 mg/kg every 6 hours for the remainder of that day and for 2 days following the procedure.

plus

Streptomycin

(as above)

For patients suspected to be allergic to the penicillins:

Erythromycin can be given (instead of penicillin or ampicillin)

For dosage and duration, see suggested prophylaxis schedule for dental procedures.

plus

Streptomycin

(as above)

Vancomycin can be given as an alternative to erythromycin

0.5 gm to 1.0 gm intravenously 1 hour prior to procedure and then 0.5 gm intravenously every 6 hours for the remainder of that day and for 2 days* following the procedure.

plus

Streptomycin

Children: 20 mg/kg 1 hour prior to procedure and then 10 mg/kg every 6 hours for the remainder of that day and for 2 days following the procedure (as above).

* or longer in the case of delayed healing

Note that in each instance the antibiotic prophylaxis is started 1 hour before the procedure and not sooner. Antibiotic administration at this time assures a high blood level of the antibiotic at the time of the bacteremia risk. It is unwise to begin antibiotics a day or two prior to the procedure; this promotes the development of organisms resistant to the antibiotic being administered.

In patients with rheumatic fever who are receiving continuous antibiotics for prophylaxis of rheumatic fever, the antibiotic should be discontinued 7 days prior to the procedure to allow normal flora to regrow. Then the recommended bacterial endocarditis prophylaxis should be initiated 1 hour before the procedure. If an emergency dental procedure is necessary in a patient with rheumatic fever, the bacterial endocarditis prophylaxis dosage should be doubled and given at the recommended intervals.

CONGESTIVE CARDIAC FAILURE

Congestive cardiac failure is the most frequent emergency problem occurring in children with cardiac disease. Among the children who develop failure, 80 percent do so in the first year of life, most commonly from congenital cardiac anomalies; of the 20 percent who develop cardiac failure after 1 year of age, in half it is related to congenital anomalies and in the other half to acquired conditions. The clinical diagnosis of congestive cardiac failure rests upon the identification of the four cardinal signs: tachycardia, tachypnea, cardiomegaly, and hepatomegaly. In addition there is often a history of poor weight gain, fatigue upon eating (dyspnea on exercise), and excessive perspiration.

Once the diagnosis of cardiac failure has been made, treatment should be initiated with a digitalis preparation.

Digoxin is the preferred drug for pediatric use. This agent has a rapid action and also a relatively fast excretion rate. It may be given orally, intramuscularly, or intravenously. Except in premature infants, the dosage is greater on a weight basis for infants than for older children. For parenteral administration, recommended digitalizing doses per kilogram of body weight of digoxin are: for premature infants, 0.03 to 0.04 mg; for children up to 2 years, 0.05 to 0.06 mg; and for children over 2 years, 0.03 to 0.04 mg.

In general usage, half of the total digitalizing dose is given initially; one fourth at 6 to 8 hours after the first dose; and the final one fourth at 6 to 8 hours following the second dose. In infants, the intravenous route is usually used. If necessary in emergency cases, three fourths of the digitalizing dosage may be given initially.

Twenty-four hours after the initial dose of digoxin, maintenance therapy is started. The recommended maintenance dose is 25 percent of the total digitalizing dose, with one half the maintenance dose given in the morning and one half in the evening. These recommendations are merely guidelines, and the dose may have to be altered according to the patient's response to therapy or the presence of digitalis toxicity. During digitalization, it is important that the patient be monitored with an electrocardiographic rhythm strip before the administration of each portion of the digitalizing dose, to detect digitalis toxicity. Alterations in the ST segments are indications of digitalis effect but *not* toxicity. Digitalis toxicity is indicated by a prolonged PR interval or cardiac arrhythmia such as nodal or ventricular premature beats. Clinical signs of digitalis toxicity are nausea, vomiting, anorexia, and lethargy.

Other therapeutic measures are useful in the treatment of children with congestive cardiac failure. Oxygen should be administered. This is most easily done during childhood with the use of a croup tent or isolette. If, following full digitalization, the infant continues to show signs of failure, the diet should be restricted in salt. Since the infant's diet is primarily milk, salt restriction can be achieved by substitution of a formula made for premature infants in which the sodium content is about 7 mEq/L.

Diuretics are also indicated in many patients with congestive cardiac failure. Although peripheral edema is uncommon in infants with cardiac failure, perhaps because they are supine much of the time, they do retain sodium and fluid. The major manifestations of edema are tachypnea and dyspnea. Lasix is the diuretic most commonly used in the acute treatment of cardiac failure and is usually given parenterally, 1 mg/kg. The oral dosage is 2 to 4 mg/kg. The effect begins promptly. With repeated use, serum sodium and potassium levels must be checked frequently.

Chlorothiazide (25 mg/kg/day) may be used for chronic long-term management of congestive cardiac failure.

Patients receiving chronic diuretic therapy may develop hypokalemia, and the low potassium enhances the development of digitalis toxicity. Potassium supplementation should be given to such patients. Older children should be encouraged to take potassium-rich foods, such as oranges, bananas, and raisins, as part of their regular diet.

Morphine (0.1 mg/kg) is extremely useful in treating the infant with major respiratory distress associated with congestive cardiac failure and the infant with pulmonary edema who is tachypneic, dyspneic, and dusky. On the other hand, it is extremely dangerous in children with underlying pulmonary disease.

Congestive cardiac failure is not a disease but a symptom complex caused by an underlying cardiac condition. After treatment of congestive cardiac failure, consideration must be given to the type of cardiac disease that produced the failure.

Operable lesions such as coarctation of the aorta or patent ductus arteriosus may have caused the cardiac failure. Therefore, following the treatment of congestive failure in any infant, appropriate angiographic and catheterization studies should be performed to establish the diagnosis. Once a diagnosis is made, one has a choice concerning management. If the infant continues to manifest problems and poor weight gain, either a palliative or a corrective procedure should be carried out. On the other hand, if the infant gains weight and does well, a conservative approach is appropriate. Since in older children congestive cardiac failure results from acquired cardiac conditions, cardiac catheterization may not be required because the etiology is often evident from history, physical examination, or laboratory findings. If appropriate, treatment should be undertaken against the cause that triggered the failure.

Conditions associated with increased pulmonary blood flow have an increased incidence of pneumonia. Pneumonia can be an event precipitating congestive cardiac failure. It should be sought in children with failure and treated appropriately if present.

CARDIOPULMONARY RESUSCITATION

Physicians caring for newborns and young infants often must treat cardiopulmonary arrest. This catastrophic event obviously requires prompt and precise treatment.

While the term "arrest" indicates cessation of respiration or cardiac action, cardiopulmonary support may also be required for infants with extremely slow or depressed cardiac and pulmonary function, to maintain normal oxygen delivery to tissues.

When a cardiac arrest occurs, help must be sought and a chain of command established for the care of the patient. In teaching hospitals, often too much help is available and a leader fails to emerge. Usually two or three physicians and two nurses are sufficient in these emergency situations. The physician with the greatest experience should direct the care and order the medications. He does not have to have his hands on the patient, but should be in a position to view the overall clinical situation.

In an arrest, a sharp blow on the chest may initiate cardiac action, but if this fails the following steps are necessary.

Airway

An adequate airway must be established. This can be accomplished without placement of an endocardial tube. Intubation is a time-consuming process that may increase vagal tone and further slow the heart. A finger should be placed in the mouth to remove any foreign matter and the head turned so the fluid material drains from the mouth. The head should then be tipped (Fig. 64) so that the nose, pharynx, and trachea form a straight line. The tongue may fall backward into the mouth and can be held against the floor of the mouth by the thumb.

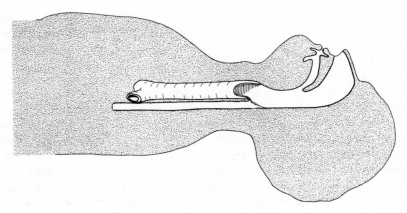

Figure 64. Proper position of head and airway for cardiopulmonary resuscitation. Airway is straightened by tipping chin up.

Breathing

Once a patent airway has been established, pulmonary resuscitative procedures begin. The child is ventilated either by a mouth-to-mouth method (older children) or a mouth-to-nose-and-mouth (infants) method. The physician's mouth is placed about the mouth or mouth and nose, forming a tight seal. The physician then in an even and unhurried way exhales into the patient at a rate of 16 times per minute. (If oxygen is available, with an Ambu bag, the advantage is obvious.)

Circulation

Once ventilation has been established, attention is directed to the circulation, and cardiac massage is begun. At a rate of 60 times per minute, the lower portion of the sternum is forcefully depressed 2 cm and released. In this way the heart is alternately compressed between the sternum and spine. Adequacy of cardiac massage can be assessed by the forcefulness of peripheral pulses.

Definitive Treatment

Once the first three steps have been undertaken, an intravenous route should be established and an electrocardiograph connected. Treatment of the invariable acidosis can be initiated, and therapy for specific electrocardiographic abnormalities can be undertaken. At this time the patient can be intubated.

Once the electrocardiograph has been placed, the underlying cardiac rhythm can be determined and appropriate therapy begun.

One of the two common types of rhythms that may appear in cardiac arrest is extreme bradycardia or asystole, the electrocardiogram appearing either as a flat line or as a slow, broad QRS complex. The purpose of treatment in such patients is to enhance rhythmicity of the heart.

Epinephrine is the first drug of choice because it enhances coronary perfusion and myocardial contraction. It can be injected into the heart or intravenously. If this does not produce normal sinus rhythm, an infusion of isoproterenol may be given. If bradycardia persists, atropine should be administered to block vagal stimulation that may be slowing the heart. These drugs can be repeated if the rhythm persists.

Ventricular tachycardia or fibrillation is the other common type of cardiac rhythm. This type of arrhythmia is related to rapid, nonsynchronized myocardial contraction, leading to ineffective cardiac output.

Ventricular tachycardia is characterized by rapid QRS complexes occurring at regular intervals, while ventricular fibrillation shows a pattern of erratic ventricular activity that in some patients is only an undulating baseline and is termed *slow fibrillation*. In other cases the complexes are deeper, and this is termed *coarse fibrillation*.

Electrical defibrillation using a DC cardioverter is the best treatment of ventricular tachycardia or fibrillation. If slow fibrillation is present, administer calcium gluconate or epinephrine intravenously in an attempt to convert the slow fibrillation to coarse fibrillation. Cardioversion can then be attempted with greater certainty of success. Usually a low dose of wattage is used initially; it can be increased if the initial effort is unsuccessful.

If the infant is still in ventricular fibrillation, either lidocaine or procainamide can be administered intravenously. Lidocaine can be repeated at 5- to 10-minute intervals if the rhythm persists.

With prolonged resuscitation and persistent acidosis, serum potassium rises and myocardial contractility decreases. Calcium gluconate may maintain the calcium-potassium ratio and improve myocardial contractility. During any infusion of calcium, the rhythm and rate must be carefully monitored.

INDEX

Acyanosis and increased pulmonary blood flow, *see* Left-to-right shunt.
Ampicillin, 190
Angiocardiography, 44
Antibiotic prophylaxis
 for adenoidectomy and bronchoscopy, 189-190
 for dental procedures and tonsillectomy, 189-190
 for gastrointestinal and genitourinary tract surgery and instrumentation, 190-191
 for surgery of infected tissues, 190-191
Aorta, coarctation of
 cardiac catheterization and angiography, 92-93
 clinical findings, summary of, 92
 electrocardiographic features, 91
 history, 90
 in neonate, 183
 natural history, 93
 operative considerations, 93
 physical examination, 90-91
 roentgenographic features, 92
 summary, 93-94
Aortic stenosis, *see* Stenosis, aortic.
Aortic valvular stenosis
 cardiac catheterization, 98
 clinical findings, summary of, 97
 electrocardiographic features, 96-97
 history, 95-96
 natural history, 98
 operative considerations, 98
 physical examination, 96
 roentgenographic features, 97
 summary of, 98

Aortography, 44
Arrhythmia(s)
 atrial, 170-172
 cardiac, 170-177
 junctional, 173
 ventricular, 173-176
Arthritis, 156
Arthralgia, 157
Asplenia syndrome, 151-152
 polysplenia, 151-152
Atrial contraction, 14
Atrial fibrillation, 172
Atrial flutter, 171-172
Atrial premature systole, 171
Atrial septal defect, 73-79
 cardiac catheterization, 79
 clinical findings, summary of, 78
 electrocardiographic features, 76-77
 history, 75
 natural history, 78-79
 operative considerations, 79
 physical examination, 76
 roentgenographic features, 77-78
 summary of, 79
Atrial sinus arrhythmia, 170-171
Atrial sinus tachycardia, 171
Atrial supraventricular tachycardia, paroxysmal, 171
Atrioventricular conduction, prolonged
 first degree heart block, 177
 second degree heart block, 177
 third degree heart block, 177
Atrioventricular conduction, shortened, 176-177
Auscultation of heart, 13-15

BLOOD pressure, 10-12
  auscultatory method, 11
  flush method, 11
  palpatory method, 11

CARDIAC arrhythmias
  conduction disturbances, 176-177
  pacemaker disturbances, 170-176
Cardiac conditions, acquired
  arrhythmias, 170-177
  endocarditis, bacterial, 165-167
  Marfan's syndrome, 167
  myocardial diseases, primary, 160-165
  pericarditis, 168-170
  prolapsing mitral valve, 167-168
  rheumatic fever, acute, 155-160
Cardiac conditions in neonate, 178-184
Cardiac examination
  auscultation of heart, 13-15
  heart sounds, 16-18
  murmur(s), 18-23
Cardiac failure, congestive, 5, 191-193
  in neonate, 181
Cardiac malformations, congenital
  left-to-right shunt, 50-85
  lesions, obstructive, 85-111
  other anomalies, 145-154
  right-to-left shunt, 111-144
Carditis, 156
Cardiopulmonary resuscitation
  airway, 193
  breathing, 194
  circulation, 194
  definitive treatment, 194-195
Catheterization, cardiac
  complications of, 43-44
  procedure, 41-43
Chorea, 156-157
Complete transposition of great arteries, 114-119
Conduction disturbances
  prolonged atrioventricular conduction, 177
  shortened atrioventricular conduction, 176-177
Congenitally corrected transposition of great arteries, 145-147
Cyanosis and diminished pulmonary blood flow, 130-144
  Ebstein's malformation, 142-144
  pulmonary atresia, 139-142
  tetralogy of Fallot, 130-135
  tricuspid atresia, 135-139

DEXTROCARDIA, 148-150
  dextroposition, 150
  dextroversion with situs solitus, 150
  situs inversus heart, 148-150

Diagnostic methods
  electrocardiography, 23-31
  history, 3-6
  physical examination, 6-23
  special diagnostic procedures, 35-44
  thoracic roentgenography, 31-35
Diet, 187-188
Discrete membranous subaortic stenosis
  cardiac catheterization, 101
  electrocardiographic features, 100
  history, 100
  natural history, 100-101
  operative considerations, 101
  physical examination, 100
  postoperative results, 101
  roentgenographic features, 100
  summary of, 101
Down's syndrome, 7
Dysplastic valve, pulmonary stenosis secondary to, 108-110
Dyspnea, 5

EBSTEIN'S malformation
  cardiac catheterization, 144
  electrocardiographic features, 143
  history, 143
  operative considerations, 144
  physical examination, 143
  roentgenographic features, 143
  summary of, 144
Echocardiography, 36-40
Ejection period, 14
Electrocardiography, 23-31
  PR interval, 26
  P wave, 25-26
  QRS complex, 26-28
  Q wave, 29
  ST segment, 29
  T wave, 29-31
  U wave, 31
Endocardial cushion defect, 79-85
  cardiac catheterization, 84
  clinical findings, summary of, 83
  electrocardiographic features, 82
  history, 81
  natural history, 83
  operative considerations, 84-85
  ostium primum, 80
  physical examination, 81-82
  roentgenographic features, 82-83
  summary of, 85
Endocardial fibroelastosis, 162
Endocarditis, bacterial, 165-167
  prophylaxis, 189
Erythema marginatum, 157
Erythromycin, 189, 190
Exercise limitations, 187

FAMILY counseling, 186-187
Fatigue, 5
Fibrillation
    atrial, 172
    ventricular, 176
Flutter, atrial, 171-172
Follow-up care, 188

GONADAL dysgenesis, *see* Turner's syndrome.
Glycogen storage disease, type II, 163

HEART, malposition of, 147-152
    asplenia syndrome, 151-152
    dextrocardia, 148-150
    levocardia, 150-151
Heart sound(s)
    first, 16
    fourth, 18
    opening snaps, 18
    second, 16
        splitting, 16
            paradoxical, 17
            wide, 17
    systolic ejection clicks, 18
    third, 17
Hematocrit determinations, 35-36
Hemodynamic principles, 45-50
Hemoglobin determinations, 35-36
Hypertension, pulmonary, 48
Hypertrophic subaortic stenosis, idiopathic, 162-163
Hypoplastic left ventricle syndrome in neonate, 181-183
Hypoxia in neonate, 183

INFECTION(S), respiratory, 5
Isovolumetric contraction period, 14
Isovolumetric relaxation period, 14

LEFT coronary artery, anomalous origin, 163-165
Left-to-right shunt, 50-85
    atrial septal defect, 73-79
    endocardial cushion defect, 79-85
    patent ductus arteriosus, 67-73
    summary of, 85
    ventricular septal defect, 51-67
Lentigo, generalized, *see* Leopard syndrome.
Leopard syndrome, 8-9
Lesion(s)
    admixture
        total anomalous pulmonary venous connection, 119-126
        persistent truncus arteriosus, 126-130
        total anomalous pulmonary venous

connection with obstruction, 123-126
        total anomalous pulmonary venous connection without obstruction, 121-123
    transposition of great arteries, complete, 114-119
    obstructive, 85-111
        aortic stenosis, 94-104
        coarctation of aorta, 88-94
        pulmonary stenosis, 104-111
Levocardia
    levoposition, 151
    levoversion of situs inversus, 150
Limb-heart syndrome(s), 9-10

MALE Turner's syndrome, *see* Noonan's syndrome.
Management and treatment
    antibiotic prophylaxis, 189-191
    bacterial endocarditis prophylaxis, 189
    cardiopulmonary resuscitation, 193-195
    congestive cardiac failure, 191-193
    diet, 187-188
    exercise limitations, 187
    family counseling, 186-187
    follow-up care, 188
    general considerations, 185-189
Marfan's syndrome, 167
Mitral valve, prolapsing, 167-168
Murmur(s)
    continuous, 20
    early diastolic, 19
    ejection systolic, 19
    functional, 21-23
        bruits in neck, 22
        cardiopulmonary, 22
        pulmonary flow, 22
        twangy string, 22
        venous hum, 22
    late diastolic, 20
    location in cardiac cycle, 19-20
    location on thorax, 20-21
        aortic area, 21
        mitral area, 21
        pulmonary area, 21
        tricuspid area, 21
    loudness of, 21
    mid-diastolic, 20
    pansystolic, 19
    pitch of, 21
    radiation of, 21
Myocardial disease(s), primary, 160-165
    endocardial fibroelastosis, 162
    hypertrophic subaortic stenosis, idiopathic, 162-163
    left coronary artery, anomalous origin, 163-165
    myocarditis, 161

Myocardial disease(s)—*continued*
  obscure origin, 161
  systemic disease, involvement with, 163
    glycogen storage disease, type II, 163
Myocarditis, 161

NEONATE, cardiac conditions in
  congenital diseases, 181-184
  physiology, 178-181
Neurologic symptoms, 6
Nodules, subcutaneous, 157
Noonan's syndrome, 8

OBSTRUCTIVE lesions, *see* Lesions, obstructive.
Ostium primum defect, 80

PACEMAKER disturbances
  atrial arrhythmias, 170-172
  junctional arrhythmias, 173
  ventricular arrhythmias, 173-176
Patent ductus arteriosus, 67-73
  clinical findings, summary of, 71-72
  electrocardiographic features, 70-71
  history, 68-69
  natural history, 72
  operative considerations, 72-73
  physical examination, 69-70
  roentgenographic features, 71
  summary of, 73
Penicillin, 189, 190
Pericarditis
  clinical and laboratory findings, 168-169
  electrocardiographic features, 169
  roentgenographic features, 169-170
  treatment, 170
Peripheral pulmonary artery stenosis
  cardiac catheterization, 110
  electrocardiographic features, 110
  history, 110
  natural history, 110
  operative considerations, 111
  physical examination, 110
  roentgenographic features, 110
Persistent truncus arteriosus, 126-130
  cardiac catheterization, 129
  clinical findings, summary of, 129
  electrocardiographic features, 128
  history, 128
  natural history, 129
  operative considerations, 129-130
  physical examination, 128
  roentgenographic features, 129
  summary of, 130
Phase reactants, acute, 157-158
Physical examination
  blood pressure, 10-12
  cardiac examination, 13-23
  infectious disease, syndrome(s) following, 10-12

syndrome(s) with familial occurrence, 8-10
syndrome(s) with gross chromosomal abnormalities, 7-8
Physiology, neonatal, 178-181
Polysplenia syndrome, 151-152
Premature beats, ventricular, 174-175
PR interval, 26
  prolonged, 157
Prophylaxis, *see* Antibiotic prophylaxis.
Pulmonary atresia, 139-142
  cardiac catheterization, 141
  clinical findings, summary of, 141
  electrocardiographic features, 141
  history, 140
  operative considerations, 141-142
  physical examination, 140
  roentgenographic features, 141
  summary of, 142
Pulmonary stenosis secondary to dysplastic valve
  cardiac catheterization, 109
  electrocardiographic features, 109
  history, 108
  natural history, 109
  operative considerations, 109-110
  physical examination, 108-109
  roentgenographic features, 109
Pulmonary valvular stenosis
  cardiac catheterization, 107
  clinical findings, summary of, 106-107
  electrocardiographic features, 106
  history, 105
  natural history, 107
  operative considerations, 108
  physical examination, 105-106
  roentgenographic features, 106
  summary of, 108
P wave
  amplitude, 25
  axis, 25
  duration, 26

QRS complex
  amplitude, 27-28
  axis, 26-27
    deviation, left, 27
    deviation, right, 27
  duration, 28
Q wave
  amplitude, 29
  duration, 29

RAPID filling phase, 14
Rheumatic fever, acute, 155-160
  criteria, major
    arthritis, 156
    carditis, 156

Rheumatic fever, criteria, major—*continued*
  chorea, 156-157
  erythema marginatum, 157
  nodules, subcutaneous, 157
  criteria, minor
    arthralgia, 157
    fever, 158
    phase reactants, 157-158
    previous history, 158
    PR interval, prolonged, 157
  long-term care, 160
  prophylaxis, 159-160
  treatment, 158
Right-to-left shunt, 111-144
  cyanosis and diminished pulmonary
    blood flow, 130-144
  lesions, admixture, 114-130
Roentgenography, thoracic, 31-35
Rubella syndrome, 10

SINUS arrhythmia, atrial, 170-171
Sinus tachycardia, atrial, 171
Situs solitus, 148
Slow filling phase, 14
Special diagnostic procedures
  angiocardiography, 44
  aortography, 44
  catheterization, cardiac, 40-44
  echocardiography, 36-40
  hemoglobin and hematocrit determi-
    nations, 35-36
Squatting, 5
Stenosis
  aortic, 94-103
    subaortic, discrete membranous, 100-101
    supravalvular, 101-103
    valvular, 95-99
  discrete membranous subaortic, 100-101
  hypertrophic subaortic, idiopathic,
    162-163
  peripheral pulmonary artery, 110-111
  pulmonary, 104-111
    peripheral pulmonary artery, 110-111
    secondary to dysplastic valve, 108-110
    valvular, 105-108
  supravalvular aortic, 101-103
  valvular pulmonary, 105-108
Streptomycin, 190
ST segment, 29
Supravalvular aortic stenosis
  cardiac catheterization, 103
  electrocardiographic features, 102-103
  history, 102
  natural history, 103
  operative considerations, 103
  physical examination, 102
  postoperative results, 103
  roentgenographic features, 103
  summary of, 103

Supravalvular aortic stenosis syndrome, 9
Supraventricular atrial tachycardia,
    paroxysmal, 171
Syndrome(s)
  asplenia, 151-152
  Down's, 7
  familial, 8-10
  hypoplastic left ventricle, in neonate,
    181-183
  leopard, 8-9
  Marfan's, 167
  Noonan's, 8
  polysplenia, 151-152
  rubella, 10
  supravalvular aortic stenosis, 9
  trisomy 18 (E), 7-8
  trisomy 13 (D₁), 8
  Turner's, 7
  with gross chromosomal abnormalities,
    7-8
Systemic disease, myocardial involvement
    in, 163
Systole, atrial premature, 171

TACHYCARDIA
  atrial sinus, 171
  atrial supraventricular, paroxysmal 171
  ventricular, 175
Tetrad spells, 132
Tetralogy of Fallot, 130-135
  cardiac catheterization, 134
  clinical findings, summary of, 133-134
  electrocardiographic features, 133
  history, 131-132
  medical management, 134-135
  natural history, 134
  operative considerations, 135
  physical examination, 132-133
  roentgenographic features, 133
  summary of, 135
Total anomalous pulmonary venous con-
    nection, 119-121
  summary of, 126
  with obstruction
    cardiac catheterization, 125-126
    clinical findings, summary of, 125
    electrocardiographic features, 125
    history, 124
    operative considerations, 126
    physical examination, 124-125
    roentgenographic features, 125
  without obstruction
    cardiac catheterization, 122
    clinical findings, summary of, 122
    electrocardiographic features, 121-122
    history, 121
    operative considerations, 123
    physical examination, 121
    roentgenographic features, 122

Total anomalous pulmonary venous connection—*continued*
  summary of, 123
Transposition of great arteries, complete, 114-119
  cardiac catheterization, 117
  clinical findings, summary of, 117
  electrocardiographic features, 116
  history, 116
  operative considerations, 118-119
  physical examination, 116
  roentgenographic features, 115-117
  summary of, 119
Transposition of great arteries, congenitally corrected, 145-147
Tricuspid atresia, 135-139
  cardiac catheterization, 139
  clinical findings, summary of, 138
  electrocardiographic features, 137-138
  history, 137
  operative considerations, 139
  physical examination, 137
  roentgenographic features, 138
  summary of, 139
Trisomy 18 (E) syndrome, 7-8
Trisomy 13 (D$_1$) syndrome, 8
Trisomy 21, *see* Down's syndrome.
Turner's syndrome, 7
T wave
  amplitude, 31
  axis, 29-30
  duration, 31

ULLRICH-Turner syndrome, *see* Noonan's syndrome.
U wave, 31
VALVULAR stenosis
  aortic, 95-99
  pulmonary, 105-108
Vancomycin, 190
Vascular ring, 152-154
Ventricular fibrillation, 176
Ventricular premature beats, 174-175
Ventricular septal defects
  large, 51-64
    cardiac catheterization, 62-64
    clinical findings, summary of, 58-59
    electrocardiographic features, 57-58
    history, 55-56
    natural history, 59-62
    operative considerations, 64
    physical examination, 56-57
    roentgenographic features, 58
  small or medium, 64-67
    cardiac catheterization, 66-67
    clinical findings, summary of, 66
    electrocardiographic features, 66
    history, 65
    natural history, 66
    operative considerations, 67
    physical examination, 65-66
    roentgenographic features, 66
    summary of, 67
Ventricular tachycardia, 175
Volume overload, in neonate, 183